DEATH AND DISEASE IN THE ANCIENT CITY

DEATH AND DISEASE IN THE ANCIENT CITY

edited by Valerie M. Hope and Eireann Marshall

London and New York

First published 2000
by Routledge
11 New Fetter Lane, London EC4P 4EE

Simultaneously published in the USA and Canada
by Routledge
29 West 35th Street, New York, NY 10001

Routledge is an imprint of the Taylor & Francis Group

Typeset in Garamond by Taylor & Francis Books Ltd
Printed and bound in Great Britain by MPG Books Ltd, Bodmin

British Library Cataloguing in Publication Data
A catalogue record for this book is available from the British Library

Library of Congress Cataloging in Publication Data
Death and disease in the ancient city / edited by Valerie M. Hope and
Eireann Marshall.
p. cm.–(Routledge classical monographs)
Includes bibliographical references and index.
1. Medicine, Greek and Roman. 2. Urban health–Rome. 3. Urban
health–Greece. I. Hope, Valerie M., 1968– II. Marshall, Eireann, 1967–
III. Series.
R138.5 .D39 2000
610'.93–dc21 99–462420

ISBN 0–415–21427–0

TO EMMANUEL AND SEBASTIAN
AND IN MEMORY OF NIA JAMES

CONTENTS

CONTRIBUTORS

John Bodel Rutgers University, New Jersey, USA

Federico Borca Università di Torino, Italy

Roger Brock University of Leeds

Valerie M. Hope Open University

Jennifer Clarke Kosak Bowdoin College, Maine, USA

Hugh Lindsay University of Newcastle, Australia

James Longrigg University of Newcastle

Eireann Marshall University of Exeter

Vivian Nutton University College London

John R. Patterson University of Cambridge

ACKNOWLEDGEMENTS

The authors would like to thank a number of individuals and institutions who made this volume possible. Above all, a special thank you should go to Fiona McHardy, without whose help this volume would not have been completed. We should also like to thank the Wellcome Foundation and the Humanities Research Board for the funds they made available both for this volume and for the conference from which the papers largely derive. As regards this conference, 'Pollution and the Ancient City', the authors would like to thank Alex Nice, who helped to organise it, as well as the University of Exeter for providing funds towards it. In addition, we are indebted to Bernard Harris for his help in shaping this volume. We would also like to express our gratitude to Ray Laurence, Chris Gill and John Wilkins for reading and commenting on the contributions. There are also a number of colleagues and friends whom we would like to thank, including Mary Harlow, David Noy and Janet Huskinson. Finally, we would like to thank our families – above all our husbands, Art and Stephen, for all the support they have given us over the years.

ABBREVIATIONS

Abbreviated references to classical works follow the conventions of the *Oxford Classical Dictionary*.

AJA	*American Journal of Archeology*
AJP	*American Journal of Philology*
BCAR	*Bulletino della commissione archeologica comunale in Roma*
BICS	*Bulletin of the Institute of Classical Studies*
CA	*Cahiers Archéologique. Fin de l'antiquité et Moyen Age*
CQ	*Classical Quarterly*
JHS	*The Journal of Hellenic Studies*
JJP	*Journal of Juristic Papyrology*
JRS	*Journal of Roman Studies*
LEC	*Les Etudes Classiques*
PCPS	*Proceedings of the Cambridge Philological Society*
REA	*Revue des Etudes Anciennes*
REL	*Revue des Etudes Latines*
TAPA	*Transactions of the American Philological Association*
WS	*Wiener Studien. Zeitschrift für Klassiche Philologie und Patristik*
ZRG	*Zeitschrift der Savigny-stiftung für Rechtgeschichte (Romanische Abteilung)*

1

INTRODUCTION

Valerie M. Hope and Eireann Marshall

> She bared her poor curst arm; and Davies, uncovering the face of the corpse, took Gertrude's hand, and held it so that her arm lay across the dead man's neck, upon a line the colour of an unripe blackberry, which surrounded it
>
> Thomas Hardy, *The Withered Arm*

To cure her ailing arm, cursed by witchcraft, Gertrude Lodge of Hardy's *The Withered Arm* was advised to place the limb upon the neck of a recently hanged man, thereby 'turning her blood' and changing her constitution. The scene unites death and disease, but in an unusual fashion. Death becomes the cure of the disease rather than disease the cause of death. Unfortunately for Gertrude the shock of discovering that the hanged man, whose death she has wished for to effect her cure, is her husband's illegitimate son, leads to her own sudden demise. Death is ultimately triumphant.

The association between death and disease in the context of the ancient city lies at the heart of this volume. Linking the topics of death and disease together, however, is not as straightforward as it may at first appear. On the one hand the connection between them is clear, and is mirrored in the general organisation of this volume: disease preceded and often led to death; the two would seem to be inextricably linked. On the other hand tracing the relationship between disease and death in the ancient world is not always straightforward. The plague of Athens, for example, was defined by the ancients as a disease that caused a great number of deaths, but in ancient discussion factors other than hygiene, medicine and germs come into play (Longrigg). Equally we can find parallels to Hardy's nineteenth-century tale, where ill-health has no medical explanation and no medical cure. In the ancient world the idea of obtaining cures from the dead was not unheard-of. The bodies of the dead, especially those who had died a violent or premature death, became imbued with special powers (Hope). Disease and death were not purely medical problems, but could be part of the world of religion, superstition and even magic. This serves to emphasise that what the modern world regards as the standard associations between disease, health, hygiene and death may not have held true in the ancient context.

The subjects of death and disease are areas of current and expanding research among ancient historians and reflect interests developed from archaeological, sociological and anthropological studies. Several recent publications on the ancient city have focused upon hygiene, disease and pollution (Grmek 1991; Scobie 1986; Parker 1983). The study of the treatment of the dead by the ancients has also produced fundamental work exploring how social structures were constructed through and by funerary rituals and how the treatment of the dead reflected attitudes to death itself (Sourvinou Inwood 1995; Bodel 1994; Morris 1992; von Hesberg 1992). The contributors here explore ways in which death and disease affected the lives of the ancients by drawing upon a wide range of textual and material evidence. The chapters address views of ancient disease causation; public and private health measures; how the natural and urban environment affected the well-being of the individual; how the city was organised to protect the health and safety of the living; how the dead were disposed of; and how the living sought protection from the polluting influence of both the diseased and the dead. Human frailty and mortality influence the structure and functioning of all societies. Questions as to how the ancients coped with their own mortality, how they sought to classify and control the causes of death, and how they treated the dying and the dead, are central to any understanding of antiquity.

The volume begins with a case study which serves as a complement to this introduction by exploring both death and disease in the context of a specific settlement (Marshall). The papers then move from disease (Brock; Kosak; Longrigg; Nutton) to death (Hope; Bodel; Lindsay) by way of considerations of how concerns about disease and death affected the urban environment, topography and organisation (Nutton; Borca; Patterson). Throughout the emphasis remains on the ancient city. Death and disease, or at least their identification and description, are largely urban phenomena. This is not deliberately to dismiss the rural. In terms of disease causation there was little differentiation between the urban and rural environment (Kosak). Yet it is on the city that our evidence focuses, and it is in general from the perspective of the urban-dweller that features of the natural environment are classed as healthy or unhealthy (Borca; Nutton). In addition, it is often only when they are viewed on a large scale that ancient death and disease become identifiable issues to a modern viewer. Bodel's estimated figures for the annual death rate in Rome emphasise that a mass population could bring into the public arena issues of how and where the dead were buried and disposed of. Equally, diseases and metaphorical diseases influenced how people viewed the urban environment and its political, social and religious organisation (Brock; Kosak). Indeed, when exploring ancient death and disease in the urban context it is often difficult to differentiate the practical and physical on the one hand from the religious and spiritual on the other. Disease and death could both be viewed as products of religious pollution (Marsall; Longrigg), but increasingly there was an awareness of the physical and hygienic implications present in disease and the importance of the proper disposal of the dead for the well-being of the city (Bodel; Lindsay). In short, death and disease, however they were defined and viewed, could become important factors in shaping the urban environment. How an ancient city was structured, functioned and was also perceived by its inhabitants was in part influenced by responses, reactions and beliefs about death and disease. Some of these had a positive impact for life in the city others less so.

Marshall investigates how both death and disease were regarded and defined in the ancient Greek city. Using the city of Cyrene as a case study Marshall notes how the dead, as a cause of pollution, were marginalised and distanced from the city. The dislocation of death helped to define the city because it defined what the city was not. However, a few prized heroes were buried at the very heart of Cyrene. Power and status could counteract pollution, and Marshall argues that this indicates that pollution was regarded as a religious issue rather than one of hygiene. Indeed disease in the city was often seen in metaphorical rather than physical terms; political disorder was often conflated with medical illness and the health of the city was perceived as the preserve of it rulers. The ancient view of disease causation and medical treatment was often closely connected to religion and the gods.

The complexity of ancient views on disease causation, and its relationship to the ancient Greek city in particular, is a theme taken up in the chapters by Longrigg, Kosak and Brock. All are interested in literary representations and descriptions of diseases, both practical and metaphorical. Kosak explores the representation of disease and disease causation in the ancient Greek city, especially in the writings of the Hippocratic authors and tragedians. The Hippocratic writers believed that the urban environment was no more unhealthy than the country because diseases were caused by the interaction of the individual with his environment rather than by contagion. As such, diseases were not perceived to be more prevalent in the densely populated cities than in the countryside around them. This was a view which could also occur in tragedy. Kosak notes how the perception of city walls as not only protecting but also enclosing the inhabitants led some writers to represent the walls in a negative fashion. Much attention was focused on the walls of cities such as Thebes and Troy, which were not always favourably perceived; by contrast tragedians did not focus on the walls of Athens. Although the focus on city walls allowed the writers to distinguish city from country, they did not describe the city as diseased and the country as healthy. Cities might be characterised as particularly prone to political or human suffering, but they were not represented as loci of disease. However, ancient authors did describe cities which suffered from civil disorder as diseased. The causes of these metaphorical diseases were not expanded upon, but they resembled a real illness since both were caused by a lack of balance and harmony.

A similar lack of balance and harmony are noted by Brock in his analysis of *stasis*, which suggests that *stasis* could be regarded in similar terms to a real disease. In other respects the parallels between the two are less well developed. Ancient writers such as Thucydides, Lucretius and Virgil describe plagues in detail whereas diseases which afflict cities suffering from *stasis* are described in only general terms. Hence *stasis*-struck cities are said to suffer from a wound or to be in some way swollen. Equally, some writers such as Thucydides suggest an awareness that real diseases may be caused by infection and contagion whereas *stasis*-illnesses are not said to be infectious. However, Brock notes that Thucydides describes the Athenian plague and the *stasis* afflicting Corcyra in similar terms; both are caused by a collapse of morality. The way *stasis*-illnesses were presented also differed between the fifth and fourth centuries BC. Fourth-century writers, especially the orators, often described *stasis*-illnesses in more moralistic terms than their predecessors since they were influenced by personal motivation, especially the desire to discredit political foes.

Longrigg draws comparisons between the way in which mythological plagues and the Athenian plague are represented in literature. Plagues in works such as the *Iliad* and *Oedipus Rex* are often attributed to a god's anger and are cured when the relevant god is placated. Since these diseases are caused by the gods they are not infectious as such, and there was little to be gained from practical hygienic measures to prevent their spread. By contrast Thucydides does not attribute the Athenian plague to divine wrath. Thucydides provides a careful description of the plague; he suggests that it may have been exacerbated by the overcrowding in the city and also implies that it may have been infectious. However, others may not have shared Thucydides' rationalistic view of the pestilence. Few practical measures seem to have been employed to prevent its spread; there were, for example, no quarantines, evacuations or proper disposals of the dead. Some appear to have believed that divine wrath was involved; Diodorus records how the Athenians purified Delos in the belief that the plague was sent by Apollo. It would seem that the rationalism present in Thucydides, and in fifth-century BC medical texts, did not necessarily reflect ordinary opinion. Many Athenians may have perceived the plague which afflicted them in similar terms to the plagues which afflicted mythical cities.

Nutton takes up the theme of the ancient view of disease causation in exploring whether medical knowledge was employed to benefit public health and improve environmental conditions, largely in the context of the Roman period. Although some writers were aware of the medical risks to be found in the dirty, polluted and corrupted city they seem to have offered little practical advice and the emphasis generally fell on the pros and cons of the natural rather than the man-made environment. The ideal was that cities, buildings and army camps should be founded in good and healthy locations. But if a patient did live in a city on a bad site it was crucial for the doctor to know what the environmental dangers were and to recommend appropriate precautions. Yet such advice was aimed very much at the individual rather than the wider community. Matters of public health were instead issues of political and social control. The doctor might advise but he lacked influence and power. Thus from the medical perspective a healthy community was made up of healthy individuals.

Borca also explores settlement organisation, but focuses on a specific environmental factor rather than more general considerations of death and disease. Proximity to a marsh, fen or bog could make a settlement potentially unhealthy. Borca investigates how these liminal areas were in theory to be avoided when founding an ancient city. Yet in practice some settlements did develop in or near marshes and this was not always viewed as a bad thing since other environmental factors could counteract the negative aspects of marsh life. In exceptional cases marshes could even provide positive advantages, giving strategic protection to vulnerable sites. There was then a certain ambivalence towards the marsh. On the one hand the marsh was a distant 'other' place, appropriate for only beasts, brigands and barbarians, and man, like the bee, was unsuited to this dirty and damp environment. On the other hand people did live alongside swamps, marshes and fens, adapting both themselves and the environment to their advantage. The swamp might be held up as a paradigm of all that was unhealthy and diseased, but people did live within these areas and accepted them rather than seeking to destroy them.

Patterson investigates the impact of environmental factors and the effects of death and disease on urban organisation. Patterson focuses on the topography of the city of Rome, especially its periphery. What boundaries surrounded the city? and what activities did they seek to exclude and control? The boundaries defined ritual, military and economic spheres of activity, but these individual boundaries were surprisingly flexible. As the city expanded its periphery was redefined and reordered. Indeed the margins of the city were not purely associated with negative activities, the burial of the dead and noxious, unhealthy industry. Instead the periphery could be an active space – aggrandised and monumentalised – as is so well illustrated by an examination of the roads, such as the Via Annia, which led from the city. When we picture the outskirts of Rome, the roads, walls and gates, it is the tombs of the dead which often spring to mind. Yet these need to be placed in a wider environment and alongside temples, arches, gardens, houses, villas and workshops. The suburb was not just characterised by negative associations such as death and disease; instead it had the potential to display honour and prestige, even if some of the more mundane and seedy activities of the area did, in the final scenario, serve to undermine any lasting sense of glory.

Marginal zones such as the marsh and cemetery often illustrate the ambivalence with which both disease and death could be regarded. Although these areas could be viewed as unhealthy and undesirable, they are often still integrated into the urban environment (Patterson; Borca). Similarly the city itself could be seen in some ways as diseased, but in other ways as no less healthy than the countryside (Nutton; Kosak; Brock). Those who practised medicine or who sought to explain disease causation could also receive a mixed response (Nutton; Longrigg). However, this sense of ambivalence is seen most clearly in the way in which the dead and those who had contact with them were treated and regarded. The dead could be viewed as pollutants, but in some cases were allowed burial within settlements (Marshall; Patterson). Above all the corpse until its disposal was halfway between the world of the living and the world of the dead; an ambivalence and uncertainty which could affect all those who came into contact with it.

This ambivalence to the dead, dying and death is explored in the chapters by Bodel and Lindsay. Bodel focuses upon the professionals involved in Roman funerals, including their role in the disposal of the unclaimed bodies of the city of Rome. Rome's annual death rate must have been in the thousands, and ensuring that all these human remains were properly disposed of was challenging. In many ways it was regarded as a practical problem rather than a spiritual or religious one. But attitudes towards undertakers and those handling the bodies of the dead could be complex. The type of work undertaken by these individuals was necessary, but also sordid and distasteful. Undertakers appear to have been shunned and despised. Was this because they were regarded as physically dirty; or were they perceived as spiritually polluted; or were they viewed as profiting at the expense of others' misfortunes? Whatever the precise reasons, it seems that funerary workers were increasingly separated from the rest of the population; a separation they shared in common with the public executioner, an actual vehicle of death. This marginalisation of undertakers and executioners reflected their roles as moderators between the world of the living and the world of the dead.

Lindsay also notes the negative attitude to funeral professionals in exploring the nature of Roman death-pollution. There often appears to have been a fear or avoidance of the dead and those who had close contact with them. In particular Lindsay examines the impact of a death upon the family involved; the taboos which affected magistrates and undertakers; the aspects of the funeral which suggest both the announcement of and purification following death-pollution; and how ideas of pollution may have influenced the locating of graves and cemeteries. It is clear that understanding what motivated fear of contamination, and whether this was regarded as spiritual or practical, is complex. This is especially so since many of the rituals and practices were anachronistic and their meaning not fully understood.

Despite all its negative connotations and its potential to pollute, the corpse was also a powerful symbol in the hands of the living, and the chapter by Hope explores how the corpse could be manipulated through either honour or abuse. The Roman ideal may have been for decent and respectable burial in a marked grave, but some were precluded from this, while others, even if they achieved it, failed to rest in peace for long. The bodies of the dead were powerful symbols to be honoured or dishonoured; corpses could be mutilated, dumped and denied burial as a way of punishing the dead for the crimes or failings of life. At the same time the corpse could also hold a certain fascination; the severed head, the crucified criminal and the dead gladiator were feasts for the eyes. For the superstitious the dead could even gain magical and therapeutic powers; to touch certain corpses was to be cured. The simultaneous fascination, fear, honour and dishonour associated with the dead created an ambivalent attitude to the cemetery. On the one hand it was a space associated with honour, ritual and respect; on the other it was perceived as the haunt of restless spirits, witches and other unsavoury characters. The ever-present dead and the fear of death, whether brought about by natural causes such as disease or by man's hand in revenge and punishment, shaped both the urban environment and the experiences of its inhabitants.

These chapters seek to explore death and disease both as related and individual phenomena. But at the outset it needs to be emphasised that these are broad subjects and that it has not been possible to explore all aspects of death and disease or all areas where they overlap and interact. The contributions are by their nature and by the nature of the volume selective. In particular they often dwell on the practical rather than the emotional or even spiritual side of the subject. In part this is dictated by the nature of our evidence and sources. It is difficult to access how people coped with disease or faced the fact of their own mortality or dealt with the emotions, suffering and bereavement brought about by death and disease. Despite these and other caveats – some of which no doubt provide ample opportunities for future research – we believe that the following chapters provide valuable insights into death and disease in the ancient city.

2

DEATH AND DISEASE IN CYRENE

A case study

Eireann Marshall

While contemporary western cities are often represented in positive terms, as centres of culture and power, they are just as frequently associated with bad health and, ultimately, death. Urban environments have largely been perceived as harbingers of disease because of the waste disposal problems which are inherent to densely populated areas and because the spread of disease is seen to be facilitated by cramped living conditions. The city has also been perceived as unhealthy because of problems associated with the disposal of the dead. Since corpses are believed to cause disease, a vicious circle is created, wherein the likelihood of disease and death is not only increased by unhealthy urban conditions but, in turn, is increased by incidents of death itself. Influenced by modern perceptions of cities, scholars have often seen ancient cities as insanitary and polluted. Most notably, Scobie (1986) and Grmek (1991) have sought to explain how the overpopulated and insanitary living conditions found in ancient urban environments increased mortality rates. However, as I hope to show, while ancient Greeks also associated cities with death and disease, they did so in entirely different ways.

In this chapter, I use classical and Hellenistic Cyrene as a case study both for exploring the strategies ancient Greeks adopted to dispose of their dead and for examining the ways in which they associated their cities with disease. I hope to show that, in common with modern western societies, the Cyrenaeans marginalised death from their city because death was seen to cause pollution. However, in contrast to modern conceptions, Cyrenaeans believed that death brought about religious and not physical pollution. In addition, I aim to show that the Cyrenaeans did not believe that urban environments were particularly conducive to disease, largely because they did not perceive illnesses as infectious. Therefore, while Cyrene, like contemporary cities, could be represented as diseased, it was frequently seen to be ill in a metaphorical rather than in a pathological sense. In addition, the diseases which ravage Cyrene sometimes derive from divine intervention. As such, they are not thought to be caused by urban conditions.

Death and the city

Death played an important role in defining Cyrene's space and identity. First, since the dead were marginalised from the city, death helped to define Cyrene's territory and boundaries. In addition, the cult of Battus and his tomb, which was located in the *agora*, was an important focus for the construction of Cyrene's identity. As such, the dead helped to define Cyrene both by being dislocated from it and by being incorporated within it. As will be seen, the apparently contradictory ways in which death defined Cyrene provide important indications for the reasons Cyrenaeans dislocated death from their city. Since the Cyrenaeans did not necessarily dispose of their dead outside their city, it is clear that they did not isolate death from Cyrene for hygienic purposes. This suggests that the Cyrenaeans did not associate death with disease in the same way as do contemporary scholars.

The marginalisation of death from Cyrene

A number of modern scholars have illustrated that ancient Greeks marginali-sed death from their cities in various ways (in particular see Kurtz and Boardman 1971; Parker 1983; Garland 1985; Sourvinou Inwood 1995). As these authors suggest, ancient Greeks isolated the dead from their cities mainly for religious reasons, in that the dead were believed to cause religious pollution. While ancient sources do not necessarily indicate what would transpire if pollution occurred, it is clear that the maintenance of religious purity was seen to be important to the well-being of cities. This is illustrated by a late fourth-century BC Cathartic Law found in Cyrene which outlines a series of regulations which had to be followed if religious purity were to be maintained. The importance of these religious regulations is evidenced by the fact that the inscription claims that these rules were established by Apollo: 'Apollo decreed that [the Cyrenaeans] should live in Libya ... observing purifications and abstinences' (*SEG* 9.72.1–3A trans. Parker). In this passage, Apollo is said both to have founded the city and to have established its religious laws. The fact that these laws are described as being decreed when the city was founded illustrates that they were central to the city.[1]

The Cathartic Law clearly demonstrates that Cyrenaeans believed death to be a pollutant. An interesting, although somewhat controversial, passage declares that 'Except for the man Battus the leader and the Tritopateres and from Onymastus the Delphian, from anywhere else, where a man died, there is not *hosia* for one who is pure' (*SEG* 9.72.22–24A trans. Parker). Although there are a number of difficulties with this passage, it suggests that tombs, apart from those mentioned, pollute priests (Parker 1983: 337–9). Another passage found in the Cathartic Law indicates that those who came into contact with the dead became polluted: 'If a woman miscarries, if it is distinguishable, they are polluted as one who has died, but if it is not distinguishable, the house itself is polluted as if from a woman in childbirth' (*SEG* 9.72.24–27B trans. Parker). This regulation stipulates that stillborn infants only caused pollution if they were fully formed, i.e. if they looked like other babies. The fact that Cyrenaeans found it necessary to distinguish babies which looked human from those which were not well developed illustrates that corpses were seen to be pollutants.

While the Cathartic Law does not expand on the death-rituals and regulations followed in Cyrene, the funerary rituals which were carried out in other Greek cities indicate that death was seen to be a pollutant. (For funerary rituals see in particular Kurtz and Boardman 1971: 142, 146–7, 150; Parker 1983: 35, 38; Garland 1985: 21–37; Burkert 1985: 79). In the first place, the dead themselves had to be cleansed and anointed. Furthermore, the relatives of the deceased were temporarily marginalised from society and needed to be ritually cleansed before they could re-enter society. In addition, vessels were placed outside of residences in which bodies had not yet been removed so that visitors could purify themselves. Houses in which people died were also ritually cleansed with seawater three days after the death occurred; the hearth and water supply were also purified. The fact that ancient Greeks established funerary rites which cleansed both people and residences which had come into contact with the dead illustrates that death was seen to cause ritual pollution (see Lindsay, in this volume, for Roman funerary rituals).

Since death was perceived to be a pollutant, it was dislocated from cities. This is emphasised by the *ekphora*, the second stage of the funerary rites carried out in most Greek cities, in which the dead were carried outside of the city in order to be buried. The Cathartic Law provides an example of how death was marginalised from Cyrene. This law prescribes that: 'If disease … or death should come against the country or the city, sacrifice in front of the gates [in front of] the shrine of aversion to Apollo Apotropaius a red he-goat' (*SEG* 9.72.4–7A trans. Parker). The fact that the shrine which protected Cyrene against death and disease was located outside the city suggests that the Cyrenaeans wanted to dislocate death from their city.

Tombs provide the most potent indication of the way in which death was marginalised from ancient cities. While tombs needed to be located near cities so that they could be properly cared for, they were normally located outside cities because they caused pollution. (For the location of tombs in ancient Greece see Kurtz and Boardman 1971: 70, 72–3, 92; Garland 1985: 93, 106; Parker 1983: 39, 42, 72–3). While the precise location of city walls can be difficult to determine, archaeological evidence suggests that tombs were almost always extramural (Parker 1983: 72–3). This is also suggested by literary sources. For example, in a well-known letter, Cicero explains that an ancient law prevented him from arranging a burial within Athens (*ad Fam.* 4.12.3).

The extramural tombs which line the main arteries of Cyrene are a visual reminder of the dislocation of death from the city. (For Cyrene's tombs see Cassels 1955; Dent 1985). It is clear that, throughout their history, Cyrenaeans invested a great deal of effort and money into tombs, apparently because tombs helped to define the status of the deceased and his family. It is probably for this reason that tombs were placed along the city's important roads. Far from being hidden away, death can be seen as a public spectacle since tombs were meant to be seen (Garland 1985: 106, 108). However, Cyrenaeans were also careful to distance this spectacle from the city by locating tombs outside the city walls.

Since it was marginalised from the city, death helped to define Cyrene's space and its boundaries. As Cyrenaeans, like other ancient Greeks, believed that death should be expelled from the city, it was necessary for them to define what lay inside and outside their city. In other words, the dislocation of death required that the city's limits be outlined. In Cyrene, as in most ancient Greek cities, it was city walls which outlined and enforced the city's boundaries. (For Cyrene's walls, see in particular Goodchild 1971; White 1998). This is indicated by the fact that Cyrenaeans placed a shrine to Apollo Apotropaius outside Cyrene's gates (*SEG* 9.72.4–7A). The fact that the Cyrenaeans dislocated death from Cyrene by placing this shrine outside their city's walls indicates that these walls marked the city's boundaries.

As they marked the city's boundaries, walls defined what belonged inside and outside the city. In doing so, walls outlined the area covered by the city and, as such, they defined urban space. Walls not only marked a city's limits but also enforced them. Therefore, walls ensured that extraneous elements were marginalised from cities. In other words, walls expelled death from cities just as they were designed to repel enemies from the city. Therefore, as Kosak illustrates elsewhere in this volume, it can be seen that walls acted like *cordons sanitaires* protecting cities from dangers coming from outside. It is, perhaps, because they defined urban space and ensured its well-being that walls came to symbolise cities. For example, in his *Hymn to Apollo*, Callimachus uses the walls of the city as a metaphor for the city itself (line 15; Williams 1978: 27).

So, the fact that death needed to be dislocated from the city meant that urban space needed to be defined. In other words, the marginalisation of death required walls both to define the city's boundaries and to expel extraneous elements, such as death, from the city. Therefore, it seems likely that extramural burials began with the formation of *poleis* or at least with the definition of the city's limits (Kurtz and Boardman 1971: 70; Burkert 1985: 191). In this way, it can be seen that the dislocation of death helped to define the city because it defined what the city was not.

The incorporation of death within the city

The Cathartic Law alludes to an apparent contradiction in the way in which

Cyrenaeans perceived their dead. While the tombs of the ordinary dead were seen to be pollutants, the tombs of heroes, such as Battus, the Tritopateres and Onymastus, were not (*SEG* 9.72.22–24A). Likewise, while most dead, including the Battiad kings who succeeded Battus, were buried outside of Cyrene, Battus and the aforementioned heroes were buried within the city (Pindar, *Pythian* 5.96–8). As such, it can be seen that death could be integrated within Cyrene. Indeed, Battus' tomb and his cult were important both for defining the city centre and for defining Cyrenaean identity.

Ancient sources represent Battus as being solely in charge of the foundation of Cyrene (Pindar, *Pythian* 4.5–8, 63; 5.87–8; Herodotus 4.150, 155–7. In the Theran version of the foundation of Cyrene, the oracle is given to Grinnus; Callimachus, *Hymn* 2.65; Diodorus 8.29; Pausanias 10.15.6; Heraclides Lembus 16 Dilts p. 20 = *FHG* II, 212; *SEG* 9.189; 9.3). It is principally through his association with Apollo, who is said to have given Battus the oracle to found the city, that Battus is represented as central to the foundation of Cyrene (Pindar, *Pythian* 4.5–6; Herodotus 4.154; Diodorus 8.29; Callimachus, *Hymn* 2.63–8; *SEG* 9.189). Although it is clear that cities were not founded by a single colonising expedition, colonies attributed the foundation of their cities to one man because this allowed them to remember and commemorate their foundations more easily (see for example Herodotus 5.42; 4.147; Pindar, *Olympian* 7.30. See also Graham 1964: 8–22 and Moggi 1983: 984–9). As a result, the founder, or *oecist*, became symbolic of the foundation and of the city's existence.

Ancient sources also credit Battus with establishing some of Cyrene's principal festivals. In his fifth *Pythian*, Pindar says that Battus both improved sanctuaries and established a road used for the festivals of Apollo (lines 89–92. For the way in which Battus is said to construct Cyrene's space see Chamoux 1953: 130; Applebaum 1979: 14; Calame 1990: 311; Giannini 1990: 83). In addition, Callimachus says that Battus erected a temple to Apollo and that he established the Carneian festival at Cyrene (*Hymn* 2.76–9. See also *SEG* 9.189). In these passages, the festivals and shrines which Battus is said to have established are dedicated to Apollo. His establishment of these honours to Apollo emphasises his link with the god. The Apolline festivals and temple were also central to Cyrene, and their association with Battus suggests that he was believed to be at the heart of the city, both physically and spiritually.

It was through his death, and in particular through the cult which centred around his tomb, that Battus was commemorated in Cyrene. Like other *oecists*, Battus was heroised after his death. This is indicated by Pindar in his fifth *Pythian* when he says that Battus: 'was blessed when he was among men and thereafter he was venerated as a hero' (lines 94–5. See also schol. *ad loc.* = Drachmann II p. 189). As a number of recent scholars have illustrated, the veneration of heroes centred on their tombs (Burkert 1985: 203, 206; Garland 1985: 88; Seaford 1994: 109, 111–12, 114, 129). As such, the worship of heroes resembled death-ritual in certain respects. For example, like all deceased people, heroes were believed to be present in their graves and, as a result, were fed and given liquid refreshments (Burkert 1985: 205; Garland 1985: 4, 110–20; Seaford 1994: 114). However, heroes differed from other deceased people in that they were believed to exercise power from their tombs. Heroes' bones, in particular, were thought to be powerful (Seaford 1994: 112–13). It is for this reason that Greek cities, at various different times, sought to retrieve heroes' remains. For example, the Spartans stole what they identified as Orestes' bones in the belief that these remains were instrumental in their fight against Tegea (Herodotus 1.68). The fact that heroes were thought to be influential only in the vicinity of their graves emphasises the importance of *heroa*, and by extension death, to hero worship (Burkert 1985: 203, 206).

While there are no known representations of Battus himself on coins, Cyrenaeans seem to have depicted his tomb on a series of coins.[2] These are Hellenistic bronzes which depict a mound surmounted by an Ionic column on their reverse (Robinson 1927: lxvii nos. 187 c–e pl. 19.4–5; xcvi. See also Jenkins 1974: 31). The fact that his tomb, rather than the *oecist* himself, is represented on coins emphasises the importance of Battus' death to the city.

The cult which centred around Battus' tomb was central to forging collective unity in Cyrene. As Burkert and Seaford have argued, hero worship both promoted social cohesion and was a focal point for the construction of collective identity (Burkert 1985: 204, 206; Seaford 1994: 111–13, 120). To a considerable extent, this derives from the function of death-ritual in uniting fellow mourners. Since the veneration of heroes resembled ordinary death-ritual, it allowed those who venerated the same hero to become, in Seaford's words, pseudo kin (Seaford 1994: 111–13, 120). As such, the worship of Battus united Cyrenaeans just as the commemoration of a deceased relative united ordinary Cyrenaean families. In other words, death was central to the integration of Cyrene.

The fact that Pindar's epinician odes were sung at Battus' tomb emphasises the fact that his *heroon* served as a focal point for Cyrenaean identity (Dougherty 1993; Calame 1990). The purpose of epinicians was not solely to glorify victorious athletes but also to glorify their native cities (Dougherty 1993: 103; 1994: 43). After all, success in Panhellenic games was perceived as a victory for both the athlete and his city. To this extent, the performance of an epinician was a kind of collective ritual. Since Battus' tomb was central to this collective ritual, it is clear that his *heroon* was both the focus of Cyrene's identity and lay at the heart of the city.

Battus' cult not only helped to forge collective cohesion in Cyrene but was also instrumental in forging Cyrenaean identity. In particular, the veneration of their founder allowed Cyrenaeans to objectify their colonial past and so helped them to define their identity. The cult of Battus emphasised the city's colonial history both by linking Cyrene to Thera, its mother city, and by helping the Cyrenaeans to signal their independence from Thera. In the first place, Battus' *heroon* helped Cyrenaeans to cement their ties with Thera since it appears to have contained Theran soil within it. However, at the same time the cult of Battus emphasised Cyrene's independence from Thera since it venerated the man who was believed to have guided settlers from Thera and to have established the city.

Battus was not only central to defining Cyrenaean identity but his tomb, like *heroa* in other cities, lay at the heart of the city. (For other examples see Herodotus 5.67; 6.38. For the location of *heroa* see Garland 1985: 88; Burkert 1985: 205–6; Seaford 1994: 112, 129). In his fifth *Pythian*, Pindar says that Battus 'lies asunder, at the far end of the agora' (line 93). In light of this description, Stucchi identified a tumulus tomb in the eastern corner of the *agora*, underneath the East Stoa, as Battus' tomb. The tumulus covers a hole in which ashes and bone fragments are buried (Stucchi 1965: 58–65; 1967: 55; 1975: 12; Bacchielli 1990: 12–21). Although several scholars, including Laronde, and Kurtz and Boardman, do not agree with this identification, the remains found in the tumulus suggest that Stucchi was right. (In particular, see Kurtz and Boardman 1971: 324 and Laronde 1987: 171–5. Previously a circular monument in the western part of the *agora* was identified as Battus' tomb. See Vitali 1932: 122; Hyslop 1945: 35; Chamoux 1953: 131. For the tomb in general see Goodchild 1971: 94–7.) The fact that this tomb appears to have been reconstructed on numerous occasions suggests that it continued to be important throughout much of the city's history.[3] Since the *heroon* was in the heart of the city and his veneration was central to Cyrene's identity, it can be argued that the tomb helped to define the *agora* as a focal point of the city. In other words, far from being dislocated from the city, death could be instrumental in determining the spatial centre of Cyrene.

So, it can be seen that Cyrenaeans perceived death in contrasting ways in that it was both expelled from the city and central to it. While the dead were ordinarily marginalised from the city by being buried outside the walls, the tomb of the city's founder lay in the heart of the city. To this extent, death helped to define Cyrene's space not only by being dislocated from the city but by defining the heart of the city. Death can also be seen to be central to Cyrene in that the cult of Battus, which was akin to death-ritual, was a focal point for uniting Cyrenaeans and for constructing their collective identity.

Reasons for the dislocation of death from ancient Greek cities

The fact that Cyrenaeans buried some people within their city while marginalising others indicates that death was seen to cause religious rather than physical pollution. After all, if the Cyrenaeans had believed that corpses caused physical pollution, they would have felt the need to dislocate all of their dead from Cyrene.

Ultimately, the apparent contradiction in Cyrene's burial practices derives from the fact that they conceptualised the dead in different ways. In Cyrene, as in other parts of the Greek world, different categories of dead people were seen to cause varying degrees of pollution (Parker 1983: 41–3; Garland 1985: 70, 78–9, 86, 95; Burkert 1985: 203, 206; Seaford 1994: 114–15, 117, 124). In particular, children were seen to cause less pollution than adults. Furthermore, ordinary adults were perceived to be pollutants while heroes were not. The regulations contained in the Cathartic Law concerning the stillborn illustrate the need to categorise the dead and suggest that different kinds of dead people cause varying degrees of pollution (*SEG* 9.72.24–27B). The fact that babies who were stillborn had to be defined as corpses before they were seen to cause pollution shows that the dead were perceived in different ways. As several scholars have argued, heroes were not thought to cause pollution because they were seen to have been beneficial to the city as a whole (Parker 1983: 43; Burkert 1985: 207; Seaford 1994: 116, 118). Heroes, such as Battus, not only benefited their cities during their lives but served to unite their cities because they were mourned by all of their citizens.[4] In contrast, apart from soldiers who died for their *poleis*, the majority of the dead were not thought to have been of service to their cities to the same extent. As a result, the ordinary dead did not unite their cities in the same way as heroes because they were mourned only by their families. Since heroes, unlike most dead, brought cohesion to their cities, they were not thought to cause pollution. It is for this reason that while most adults were buried outside the city walls, heroes could be buried within cities. Since all corpses are potentially physically noxious, the ancient Greek tendency to perceive some dead as more polluted than others indicates that they believed that corpses caused religious rather than physical pollution.

Since death was not seen to cause physical pollution, it is evident that it was not dislocated from the city for hygienic purposes. If the Cyrenaeans had wanted to dislocate the living from the dead for reasons of health, burying the dead in secluded parts of the city would have sufficed (Parker 1983: 72). In other words, they did not need to inhume the dead outside their city walls in order to maintain a hygienic distance between the living and the dead. After all, walls do not physically stop the spread of disease. Since walls are imaginary boundaries rather than actually being *cordons sanitaires*, it is evident that the Cyrenaeans buried their dead outside their city walls for ritualistic purposes, i.e. because the dead were believed to cause religious pollution.

In addition, ancient Greeks did not cleanse dead bodies, houses which witnessed death and those who came into contact with corpses for hygienic purposes (Parker 1983: 56–9, 226–9; Garland 1985: 6). While some cleansing rites, such as cleansing houses with sea water, may in reality have had hygienic effects, their main purpose was to restore ritual purity. If the aim of lustrations had ultimately been hygienic, ancient Greeks could have cleansed houses with ordinary water rather than sea water. As such, it can be seen that Cyrenaeans, like other ancient Greeks, did not feel the need to purify bodies in order to stop the spread of disease.

The fact that death was not seen to cause physical pollution indicates that ancient Greeks did not believe that corpses caused disease. However, ancient concepts of religious pollution resemble modern concepts of disease in several ways (Parker 1983: 218–20). In particular, while ancient Greeks did not necessarily perceive diseases as infectious, they thought that religious pollution could be spread to other people. It is for this reason that polluted people rather than diseased people were isolated from the rest of society. To this extent, it can be argued that ancient Greeks associated death with ritual pollution in a similar way to that in which modern scholars might associate death with disease.

Disease and city

The diseased city: Cyrene and civic order

Although both ancient and modern writers associate ancient cities with disease, they do so in diverging ways. While modern authors such as Grmek perceive urban environments to be conducive to contagious diseases, ancient authors frequently describe cities as metaphorically rather than physically ill. In doing so, ancient writers do not tend to explain the causes of these diseases and do not see these illnesses as being caused by pathogens.

As Brock has illustrated elsewhere in this volume, ancient sources often represent cities as patients which become ill and need to be healed. In particular, cities which suffer from *staseis* are described as physically sick. By extension, cities in which civic harmony is restored are described as being healed. Furthermore, just as cities are described as patients, those gods and rulers who restore peace to cities are represented as doctors. Therefore, although ancient writers may represent cities as metaphorically ill, they tend to describe them suffering from medical illnesses and being cured by medical remedies.

When Pindar refers to the *stasis* Cyrene suffered under Arcesilas IV, he describes the city as sick. In particular, in his fourth *Pythian* Pindar says that one needs to apply a gentle hand while caring for a festering wound (line 271). It becomes clear in the succeeding lines that Pindar describes Cyrene itself as injured since he says that it is easy even for the weak to shake a city to the ground but it is difficult to put a city back on its feet (*Pythian* 4.272–3). By describing Cyrene as ill, Pindar conflates political disorder with medical illness.

Pindar not only perceives *stasis* as an illness but also describes those who rule Cyrene and who are responsible for restoring civic order as doctors. In his fourth *Pythian*, Pindar addresses Arcesilas IV by saying 'You, Arcesilas, are a most fit doctor (*iatēr epikairotatos*) and Paian honours the light that shines from you' (line 270). In the lines which follow this passage, Pindar explains that Arcesilas must heal his ailing city (*Pythian* 4.271–4). In doing so, Pindar represents a king who brings social harmony to a city suffering from *stasis* as a doctor who cures a patient. Conversely, Parker has shown that, in other contexts, magistrates who are thought to govern badly are sometimes thought to bring various afflictions to their cities (Parker 1983: 268; Grmek 1991: 16). Therefore, ancient texts can represent those who govern well as bringing health to their cities while depicting those who misrule as harbingers of disease. The way in which ancient authors equate governing with healing indicates that they perceive cities as patients whose health is the preserve of its rulers.

Pindar also represents Apollo as a doctor who might restore Cyrene's health. Indeed, it is partly because of his connection with Apollo that Pindar represents Arcesilas IV as a healer.[5] Pindar not only says that Paian, or Apollo, assists Arcesilas but says that rulers need the help of a god if they are to restore order to their cities (*Pythian* 4.270, 274). Apollo is described as central to Cyrene's recuperation both because he was responsible for the foundation of the city and because he is a medical god. The way in which Pindar conflates these two roles, namely Apollo's establishment of cities and healing, gives a further indication of how governing is represented in terms of curing.

Throughout his fourth and fifth *Pythian* odes, Pindar describes Apollo both as the founder of Cyrene and as a god of medicine. In his fourth *Pythian*, Pindar says that Apollo brought the Theran settlers to Libya (line 259). Likewise, in his fifth *Pythian*, Pindar describes Apollo as Cyrene's *archegetes*, or founder, and says that he instilled fear into lions who threatened Battus in order that his oracle would be fulfilled (lines 60–2). Pindar also emphasises Apollo's role as a god of medicine in both of these epinicians. In his fifth *Pythian* (lines 90–1), he says that Apollo's festivals protect humanity (*Apolloniais aleximbrotois*). Although he does not describe the kind of protection Apollo offers, it seems likely that Pindar is alluding to the apotropaic functions which are attributed to Apollo in the Cathartic Law, where he is said to ward off disease and death (*SEG* 9.72.4–7). Pindar more specifically describes Apollo as a god of medicine when he says that Apollo gives men and women antidotes for serious illnesses (*Pythian* 5.63–4).

Pindar implicitly associates Apollo's role as a doctor with his role as a god of law and order by linking his practice of prescribing medical remedies with his practice of giving law to cities. Shortly after saying that Apollo gives remedies to people, Pindar says that the god gives humanity the love of law, which is antithetical to strife (*Pythian* 5.66–7). In doing so, Pindar describes law as an antidote for strife in the same way as he describes medicine as an antidote for diseases. As such, Pindar can be seen to infer that

Apollo could cure Cyrene's *stasis* with the establishment of law in the same way as he cures diseases with medicine. Apollo the doctor is, thereby, conflated with Apollo the lawgiver.

In his *Hymn to Apollo*, Callimachus also describes Apollo as a doctor and as a founder of cities. The poet refers to Apollo's healing qualities by saying that the god brings the art of medicine to doctors (Callimachus, *Hymn* 2.45–6). Callimachus more frequently emphasises Apollo's role in the founding of cities. He says that Apollo delights in founding cities and describes the god as guiding men when they establish cities (Callimachus, *Hymn* 2.55–7). Callimachus also says that Apollo, disguised as a raven, led the Theran settlers to Cyrene (*Hymn* 2.65–8).[6] In addition, Callimachus represents Apollo as guaranteeing civic order as well as founding cities. As has been seen, he describes Apollo as being responsible for ensuring that city walls remain standing (Callimachus, *Hymn* 2.15). Since Callimachus uses the walls of the city as a metaphor for the city itself, he means that the god ensures that cities are free from civil strife (Williams 1978: 27).

Callimachus explicitly represents Apollo's role in maintaining civic order in terms of him providing cities with medical remedies. In an intriguing passage, Callimachus says that Apollo's 'hair trickles fragrant oils on the ground; his hair does not drip fat but panacea. In those cities where these dews fall on the ground, all things become unharmed' (*Hymn* 2.38–41). In this passage, panacea could be seen either as the goddess Panacea or as a herb (Williams 1978: 44). However, the fact that Callimachus describes this panacea as springing from the ground suggests that it is a plant. While several medicinal herbs were described as *panaces*, it is possible that Callimachus may be referring to silphium, the famed Cyrenaican plant which was used for a number of different medical purposes and which appears to have been described as a panacea.[7] Whether this panacea is silphium or another herb, Callimachus describes Apollo as protecting cities by giving them a medical remedy. Interestingly enough, Callimachus does not say that Apollo's panacea prevents diseases but rather says that it shields cities from harm. This suggests that Callimachus viewed this herb as protecting cities from metaphorical dangers such as civil strife. Therefore, Apollo could be seen as ensuring civic order through medical means. As such, Callimachus, like Pindar, appears to equate social order with health and appears to suggest that cities can be protected from political disorder with medical remedies. Cities thereby become patients, and lawgivers become doctors.

This analysis of the way in which ancient writers link civic order and disease suggests that they associate cities with disease in a different way from modern authors. Pindar describes strife-ridden Cyrene as physically ill and represents those who might restore order to the city as doctors. Similarly, Callimachus depicts Apollo as a doctor who maintains social order with a medicinal herb. However, although Pindar depicts Cyrene as physically ill, the disease which the city suffered under its last king, Arcesilas IV, was metaphorical rather than pathological. As such, this disease was not caused by pathogens and did not bring about the death of individuals. For these reasons, this illness differs from the infectious diseases and epidemics normally associated with cities in modern analyses.

Ancient and modern writers associate cities with disease in diverging ways because they conceive of illnesses in different ways. While Thucydides (2.51.5–6) apparently links the outbreak of the Athenian plague with overcrowded conditions (see Longrigg, in this volume), ancient writers do not tend to view diseases as more prevalent in cities. Conversely, Grmek, who offers the most coherent and accessible account of disease in ancient Greece, associates ancient cities with disease because he views urban conditions as particularly conducive to disease. In particular, he argues that the disposal of waste and sewage becomes problematic in cities; as such, diseases caused by parasites, viruses and intestinal worms tend to be more common in cities (Grmek 1991: 88–90, 92). While Grmek is certainly right to argue that urban environments encourage the spread of disease, his perception of the way diseases function and the way he associates cities with illnesses is alien to ancient thought. Ancient writers largely do not see diseases as contagious and, as such, tend not to link hygiene or overcrowded conditions with illnesses (Parker 1983: 219–20). In addition, ancient texts tend to focus on cures for diseases rather than on their causes, perhaps because they do not view illnesses as contagious. Therefore, Pindar does not explain what caused the metaphorical illness which Cyrene suffered under Arcesilas IV. He does not perceive this *stasis* as causing Cyrene's disease but rather equates *stasis* with disease. Furthermore, although Pindar associates Apollo with civic order, he does not suggest that Apollo sent this illness to the Cyrenaeans because they transgressed divine law.[8] He also does not indicate which man or group of men may have caused this *stasis*/disease.

Therefore, it can be seen that when ancient writers represent cities suffering from *stasis* as medically ill, they conceive of this urban disease in a different way from modern scholars. This *stasis*/disease differs from illnesses which contemporary scholars might associate with cities in that it is not contagious and endangering the health of individuals. This suggests that ancient writers do not necessarily view disease as causing death, just as they do not see death as causing disease.

Illness and the foundation of Cyrene: epidemics and urban environments

When cities are described as suffering from pathological illnesses, the causes and antidotes for these diseases sometimes differ from those which might be offered in modern analyses. Herodotus says that Thera suffered from a drought because the city was reluctant to send a colonising expedition to Cyrene.

Herodotus' account of this drought differs from Pindar's description of the *stasis*/illness suffered under Arcesilas IV in that Herodotus does explain the cause of the drought suffered by the Therans. However, Herodotus' description of this natural disaster and its associated illnesses differs from one which might be expected from modern analysts since instead of exploring environmental and physical factors he focuses on divine intervention.

According to Herodotus, the Delphic oracle instructed either Grinnus or Battus to found Cyrene, although neither had previously intended to colonise Libya (4.150, 155). The Therans initially decided to ignore the oracle, largely because they did not know where Libya was (Herodotus 4.150). As a result, Thera suffered from a drought which lasted seven years (Herodotus 4.151).

Although Herodotus does not describe the island as suffering from a disease, ancient texts often associate droughts and excessive heat with pestilence. For example, Strabo says that the scarcity of rain in the desert regions of Libya and Aethiopia causes plagues (Strabo 17.3.10, p. 830). In addition, Apollonius and Callimachus implicitly associate droughts with plagues when they say that Ceos suffered from a pestilence after Sirius scorched the island. Since Callimachus says that Aristaeus freed Ceos of this pestilence in his capacity as the god of moisture, it is apparent that he linked the plague not only with heat but also with the lack of water (Apollonius Rhodius 2.516–27; Callimachus, *Aeitia* 75.ll.34). Therefore, it is possible that Herodotus may have viewed Thera as suffering not only from drought but also from diseases caused by droughts.

In this case, it appears that he perceived the causes of pestilences in different terms from modern scholars. Herodotus explicitly says that the drought was caused by the Therans' defiance of the Delphic oracle and implies that this drought only ended when the Therans finally sent a colonising expedition to Libya (4.150–1). By implication, it is Apollo who caused the drought and the misfortunes which may have been associated with it.

Herodotus emphasises that Thera's drought was reversed after the colonisation of Libya by describing Cyrene as being well watered. As such, the same Therans who suffered from a drought before they went to Libya enjoyed an abundance of water when they finally founded Cyrene. Indeed, the Therans are said to have chosen the site of Cyrene because of its spring and plentiful rainfall. Herodotus says that the Libyans who led the Theran settlers to Cyrene went directly to the spring of Apollo and said 'you will like it here because the sky has a hole in it' (4.158).[9] The fact that the spring was known as the Spring of Apollo may also be significant. The god who denied the Therans water when his orders were not followed can be seen to have given them water once they did follow his orders.

The fact that Herodotus attributes Thera's drought and its related diseases to Apollo indicates that he perceives the causes of plagues in different terms from modern scholars. Contemporary analysts, such as Grmek, argue that plagues are particularly prevalent in urban environments and are caused by pathogens rather than by divine retribution. In particular, Grmek argues that viral illnesses such as smallpox, mumps and measles, which are contagious but either kill or immunise their hosts, only thrive in densely populated areas (Grmek 1991: 98). Conversely, ancient authors do not tend to associate epidemics with urban conditions, largely because they do not appear to view diseases as contagious. Instead, they are more likely to believe that pestilences are caused by divine retribution. Although they do not believe that ritual infractions are always punished by gods, ancient writers sometimes perceive plagues as being sent by gods (Parker 1983: 251). For example, Diodorus believed that the Athenian plague was caused by the ritual polluting of Delos (12.58.6–7. See Longrigg, in this volume).

The way in which Herodotus describes Thera being cured from this drought illustrates how ancient and modern scholars view diseases in diverging ways. Although he appears to say that the island suffered from a pestilence, Herodotus does not depict Apollo curing Thera in medical terms. Instead, the god restores health to the island when his instructions are followed. Ancient sources describe Apollo as preventing diseases both through medical antidotes and by being appeased and venerated. While Callimachus says that Apollo prevents diseases with medical herbs, Pindar describes the god protecting humanity through his religious festivals (*Hymn* 2.38–41; *Pythian* 5.90–1). Likewise, the Cathartic Law prescribes that dedications should be made to Apollo if disease were to be prevented (*SEG* 9.72.4–7). The way in which these texts see diseases as being cured or prevented through both religious and medical antidotes suggests that ancient and modern analysts perceive illnesses to be assuaged in diverging manners. As Parker has demonstrated, ancient writers can blur the boundaries separating medical and religious cures because gods are sometimes thought to cause illnesses (Parker 1983: 207–10, 213–15). When gods are deemed to be responsible for causing diseases, patients could be cured through religious purification; this allowed relations between the patient and relevant god to be restored (Parker 1983: 213–17). The fact that there was not always a discernible difference between medical and religious prescriptions illustrates how different ancient and modern concepts of medical cures are. Ancient writers do not necessarily view diseases as being alleviated by medical remedies just as they do not always view illnesses as being caused by pathogens.

Conclusion

This analysis of classical and Hellenistic Cyrene has shown that Cyrenaeans associated their city with death and disease in ways which are alien to twentieth-century thought. First, while both ancient and modern societies associate death with pollution, they do so in differing ways in that the former believed that corpses caused ritual not physical pollution. This is emphasised by Cyrenaean burial practices and by the way in which Cyrenaeans conceptualised the dead. Had the Cyrenaeans buried their dead outside of Cyrene for hygienic purposes, they would have inhumed all corpses outside of the city walls. Likewise, if they believed that the dead caused physical pollution, they would have seen all corpses as being noxious. However, the burial of certain corpses within the city indicates that the Cyrenaeans did not believe that corpses *per se* were unhygienic and did not link death with disease in the same way as modern analysts.

In addition, although both ancient and modern analysts associate cities with disease, they do so in differing ways. First, the diseases which ancient writers associate with Cyrene are sometimes different from illnesses linked to urban centres in contemporary societies. While Pindar describes strife-torn Cyrene as medically ill, this disease is metaphorical rather than pathological. Furthermore, ancient sources can explain the causes of diseases in different ways. As has been seen, Herodotus attributes the drought suffered by the Therans, and by extension diseases which may have accompanied it, to divine intervention rather than noxious urban environments. Since ancient writers tend not to perceive illnesses as being contagious, they would not have attributed diseases to the overcrowded conditions or to the waste disposal problems inherent in most cities.

NOTES

1 Parker (1983: 334) rightly argues that it is unlikely that the Cathartic Law was a faithful transcription of an archaic law. However, this does not mean that some of the regulations contained in the decree were not archaic or, more importantly, that fourth-century BC Cyrenaeans themselves did not believe that these religious regulations were not ancient.

2 There are not many representations of Battus on coins or statues. Stucchi (1967: 113) identified Battus on a second-century AD figured capital from the House of Jason Magnus. The identification is based on the fact that silphium is represented alongside this figure. According to a scholiast to Aristophanes, *Wealth* 925 = Aristotle fr. 528, Battus was given silphium by the city. Stucchi also argued that the figure's severe hairstyle indicates that it is a copy or a variation of an archaic portrait. However, since no other portraits of the oecist exist, this identification must remain uncertain. Mingazzini (1966: 87–8) identified this figure as Oedipus.

3 Several inscriptions suggest that the *oecist* continued to be important to Cyrenaeans in the Roman period. An inscription commemorating the restoration of the temple of Apollo after the Jewish Revolt recalled Battus' erstwhile construction of this temple (*SEG* 9.189). Furthermore, an inscription from the reign of Augustus refers to Cyrene as the city of the descendants of Battus (*SEG* 9.63).

4 Nevertheless, it should be emphasised that heroes were not necessarily represented in a positive light. For example, according to one tradition, Battus spied on women carrying out the rites of the Thesmophoria in order to learn the mysteries of Demeter. When these women noticed him, they launched themselves against him and castrated him. For this myth see Suidas s.v. 'Thesmophoros' and 'Sphaktriai'. Cf. also Vitali 1932: 70 no. 185.

5 The Battiads are frequently associated with Apollo. Pindar, *Pythian* 4.260–1 says that Apollo ordained that the Battiads rule over Cyrene. Similarly, Callimachus, *Hymn* 2.68 says that Apollo promised the Battiads a walled city. Callimachus also links the Battiads with Apollo in *Hymn* 2.26–7, 67–8, 95–6. See also Herodotus 4.155, 157 for the Delphic oracle making Battus king and Herodotus 4.163 for Apollo granting kingship to eight generations of Battiads. Finally, see Diodorus 8.29, in which Apollo gave an oath to the Battiads that they would remain in power for eight generations.

6 Callimachus, *Hymn* 2.94–5 also says that Apollo blessed no other city as much as he blessed Cyrene because of his union with the nymph Cyrene.

7 For medicinal herbs being referred to as *panaces* see, for example, Dioscorides 3.48. For silphium's medical properties see Pliny the Elder, *Natural History* 22.100–7, who says that silphium was used as a purgative and diuretic. Although he wrote several centuries after Callimachus, Pliny largely based his description of silphium on Theophrastus. The fact that *laserpicium*, the Latin word for silphium, is sometimes referred to as *panaces Cheironeion*, suggests that silphium was described as a panacea. See Thraemer, in Roscher, *Mythol. Lex.* iii s.v. 'Panakeia' cc. 1482–4. Parisi Presicce (1994: 93–4) argues that silphium was known as a panacea on the basis that the *panaces Cheironeion* were also known as *laserpicium*. This panacea is also linked to silphium by virtue of the fact that Cheiron is said to have taught Aristaeus, the discoverer of silphium, the arts of healing. For example, see Apollonius of Rhodes 2.502.

8 Parker (1983: 45, 216–18, 239–40, 242–9) argues that although gods are sometimes seen to send diseases when humans transgress divine laws, infractions do not normally result in divinely sent diseases.

9 Callimachus, *Hymn* 2.88–9 also implies that this spring, or *cyra*, was the first point of embarkation for the Theran colonists. Pindar, *Pythian* 4.294 alludes to this spring when he says that the exiled Damophilus anxiously awaits the day when he could return to his city where he would enjoy a banquet near Apollo's fountain. The way in which Pindar uses this spring as a landmark emphasises its centrality to Cyrene. The importance of this spring to Cyrene can also be gauged by the fact that it was believed to be one of the derivations of the city's name. For the etymology of the city's name see Stephanus of Byzantium s.v. 'Cyrene', and Eustathius, *Paraphrase of Dionysius Periegetes*, *GGM* II p. 213. For modern commentators see Chamoux 1953: 126 and Dougherty 1993: 147. Pindar, *Pythian* 4.52–3 emphasises that Cyrene was known for its rainfall when he refers to the Cyrenaean *chora* as plains which are cloaked by a dark cloud.

3

SICKNESS IN THE BODY POLITIC

Medical imagery in the Greek polis

Roger Brock

Beset by sickness and death in reality, the cities of ancient Greece were also subject to a range of symbolic and metaphorical diseases, amongst them the equation of disorder in the state with a sickness of the body politic. This image, though not part of the Homeric repertoire, appears in Greek literature with Solon and Theognis, and seems to have become something of a commonplace as well as a staple of political discourse, to judge from the way it is parodied by Aristophanes.[1] As a widespread and substantial development of the concept of disease, the phenomenon merits investigation here in its own right.

Given the contemporary development of medical theory and practice in Greece in the fifth century BC, one would expect to observe some degree of correspondence between medical reality and medical image. In fact, what is striking is the lack of much of the medical detail one might expect to find. Likewise, there are significant divergences from the manner in which medical imagery is deployed in the modern world, a phenomenon discussed in a most illuminating way by Susan Sontag (1979; 1989). Equally, however, it does not seem to me that the image of the sickness of *stasis*, despite its considerable degree of conventionality, is to be dismissed as a dead metaphor, and in what follows, I shall argue that the central concept underlying it retains both a significant relationship to contemporary medical ideas and a genuine vitality and validity. What I want to do is, first, to draw attention to significant divergences from contemporary Greek medicine, second, to say a little about Plato's use of medical imagery, which seems to me to be the foundation of the later use of such images but rather out of line with earlier Greek usage, and finally, to argue for the real medical significance which I believe I can see in that other usage.

I

One striking feature of the image is that the disease (*nosos*) of *stasis* is not any disease in particular, in contrast to the modern usage of allusions to specific maladies such as tuberculosis, cancer and AIDS described by Sontag. In one sense, this is not surprising at all, since classical Greek doctors apparently did not identify and name as such any infectious disease. What is more striking is that the disease of civil strife has no aetiology and few, if any, symptoms. Apart from *helkos* ('wound' or 'ulcer'), which appears as an alternative term, or perhaps a precursor, to *nosos* ('disease') in the earliest instances of the image in Solon and Theognis (n. 1 above; cf. also Pi. *Pyth.* 4.271), the only specific symptoms associated with the political disease are swelling (*oidein*) in Herodotus 3.76.2 and 127.1, applied to political upheaval, and Theognis' description of an atmosphere of foreboding and uncertainty in Megara in terms of pregnancy: 'this city is pregnant, and I fear that it may beget a man to set things straight' (39–40). If anything, then, the tendency is for the image to become *more* general from the sixth to the fifth century; in the fourth, Plato and Demosthenes add to the register of symptoms inflammation, swelling, fracture and sprain,[2] but this is still hardly a great haul.

Equally striking is the absence from the medical metaphor of any anatomical detail: the body politic is articulated only to the extent of distinguishing the head, as seat of authority, from the rest of the body. Thus, an oracle allegedly given to the Argives shortly before Xerxes' invasion (Hdt. 7.148.3) distinguishes between the body and the head: 'hated by your neighbours, dear to the immortal gods, sit on your guard, holding your spear drawn in and guard the head, for the head will save the body'. How and Wells (1912) *ad loc.* identify the head with the remnant of the ruling class, which had suffered at the hands of Cleomenes at the battle of Sepeia, the body being the mass of the population, including the so-called slaves. Another oracle given to the Athenians about the same time (Hdt. 7.104.1) itemises the parts of the body in the same Homeric vocabulary, though without any specific political reference. In the same way, the nocturnal council of Plato's *Laws* is the intellect of the state, which the junior guardians serve as sense-organs (964d–5b) and, by inversion, the head governs the microcosm of the body in the *Timaeus* (69de, 70b; cf. *Laws* 942e; in Arist. *Part. An.* 670a26 the head is an acropolis). It might be held that the reference in an oracle given to the Spartans to a 'lame kingship' (*tēn chōlēn basileian*; Xen. *HG* 3.3.3) should furnish the body politic with legs, but Lysander's interpretation, that the lameness of which the Spartans were warned referred to a general dysfunction of the monarchy, is supported by other examples of *chōleuō* (*LSJ* s.v. 2) and *chōlos* (*LSJ* s.v. II) in this very broad sense.[3] In fact, the phrase *to tēs poleōs sōma* ('the body of the state') does not actually appear until the later fourth century, in Deinarchus (1.110) and Hypereides (5 col. 25), both in prosecutions of Demosthenes, perhaps not coincidentally, by which time other orators have already attributed a soul to the city, either its constitution or its laws (Isocrates 7.14, 12.138; Demosthenes fr. 13).[4] The lack of anatomical detail is not the result of ignorance, since a basic knowledge of anatomy is already reflected in Homer's descriptions of wounds in the *Iliad* (even if little advance was made thereafter until the application of dissection in the early Hellenistic period); it must therefore be a matter of deliberate choice.

Vagueness about anatomical and clinical particulars is paralleled by the very general language in which the disease of civil strife is described. To the symptomatic terms which I have already mentioned, we can add *arrōstia* of illness in general, *katabolē ... astheneias* and *prosistasthai* in the sense of 'attacks' of disease, and *sathros* ('unsound'), *hupoulos* ('festering') and (perhaps) *eklelusthai* ('be faint, fail') of conditions of sickness.[5] None of these words can really be considered technical; even the language of Thucydides' description of the Plague of Athens, though it is now generally conceded that, in Adam Parry's words (1969: 113) it 'is not entirely, is not even largely, technical', is a great deal more varied and circumstantial.

Indeed, a wider comparison between accounts of the sickness of *stasis* and the literary genre of the plague description is instructive. In examples of the latter such as those in Thucydides, Lucretius and Virgil, the enumeration of the many forms and symptoms of the disease serves to reinforce the impression of its intractability, both rhetorically, by an overwhelming enumeration of details and, in a more explicit manner, by creating an impression of an enemy too versatile and cunning for its human opponents to master; one might compare modern presentations of viral mutation or the development of 'super-bacteria' resistant to all antibiotics. In contrast, the bare assertion in the imagery that the city is sick simply establishes the existence of the disease, leaving scope for the possibility of a more hopeful prognosis. Furthermore, literary plagues are epidemics which strike a whole community, passing by contagion or infection from one individual to another – and indeed sometimes from species to species – but this dynamic is absent from the imagery, which is only concerned with the presence of the disease within the single organism of the body politic.

A comparison with a short passage from the fifth-century Hippocratic corpus (*Epidemics* 1.2), chosen more or less at random, will help to emphasise the contrast between disease in imagery and its real counterpart:

> In the majority of cases, the symptoms were these: fever [*puretoi*] with shivering, continuous, acute, not completely intermitting, but of the semitertian [*hēmitritaios*] type; remitting on one day, they were exacerbated on the next, becoming on the whole more acute. Sweats were continual, but not all over the body. Severe chill in the extremities, which with difficulty recovered their warmth. Bowels disordered, with bilious, scanty, unmixed [*akrētoisi*], thin, smarting stools, causing the patient to get up often. Urine either thin, colourless, uncococted [*apepta*] and scanty, or thick and with a slight deposit, not settling favourably, but with a crude and unfavourable deposit. The patients frequently coughed up small, concocted [*pepona*] sputa,

> brought up little by little with difficulty. Those exhibiting the symptoms in their most violent form showed no concoction [*pepasmenon*] at all, but continued spitting crude [*ōma*] sputa. In the majority of these cases the throat was throughout painful from the beginning, being red and inflamed. Fluxes slight, thin, pungent. Patients quickly wasted away and grew worse, being throughout averse to all food and experiencing no thirst. Delirium in many cases as death approached. Such were the symptoms of the consumption.
>
> (tr. W. H. S. Jones [Loeb])

In this account the disease is described in great symptomatic detail conveyed through a language of fairly dense technicality quite unlike the bare diagnosis of disease in sickness imagery. There is of course a wide disparity between the objectives of the two sorts of writing, but Thucydides' occupation of a mid-point between them in terms of expression indicates that they did not simply represent mutually exclusive choices, and recent discussions of the historian's language (Parry 1969; Hornblower 1987: 97) have tended to suggest that his restraint was an artistic rather than a practical choice.

II

I now turn from examining the descriptive qualities of medical imagery to consider its implications, which are more closely linked to the other side of the medical coin, that is, the issue of treatment. Here I shall begin with Plato and work backwards, partly because his attitudes are fairly obvious and uncontroversial, and partly because they are much more in line with later usage of this sort of imagery (well discussed in Sontag 1979: ch. 9). I should admit that my account will be rather summary, and that I shall duck completely the broader issues of the political analogy in the *Republic* and of Plato's use of parallel and reflexive corporal images of microcosm and macrocosm.

Plato's medical imagery is based on two basic concepts: the idea of health or dysfunction within an organic unity, and the equation of those in political authority with doctors, an example of Plato's fondness for craft analogies to describe the practice of philosophical statecraft (*Polit.* 297e, *Laws* 905e); that it is particularly dear to his heart is suggested by the close correspondence between passages in the *Republic* (425e–6c) and the *Seventh Letter* (330c–331a) which compare the Athenian democracy to a patient whom it is pointless to treat until he changes his way of life; in the *Seventh Letter*, the image is used to justify Plato's own refusal to intervene in Athenian politics.

This field of imagery offers Plato a number of advantages in presenting his programme. Health is a universally recognised good, and therefore rhetorically persuasive; however, it is not universally understood, and the layman would therefore be well advised to submit to the judgement of the expert, not only as to what constitutes health, but also as to the most appropriate therapy for any given malady. Finally, since the good of the organism as a whole is what matters, it is reasonable to submit parts of the body to painful processes, or even to remove them altogether, if that is what is required to restore health. Medical imagery thus adds to the general claim of the craft analogies to superior wisdom and expertise a charter for intervention which the persuasive force of the concept of health makes it hard to resist, and against which the idea of a living organism (with unspoken overtones of a finite lifespan) makes it difficult to temporise. This is true whether it is the maintenance or the restoration of health which is at issue: at times, as in the *Gorgias* (464b), Plato distinguishes the former as the province of the trainer, but in the real world of flawed constitutions it is the doctor who is much more likely to be needed. However, as we have just seen, Plato knew from personal experience that he would not necessarily be called on, and similarly in the *Gorgias* (521e–2a) he makes Socrates the true legislator identify himself with a doctor victimised by a pandering confectioner.

While the patient is expected to seek out the doctor (*Rep.* 489 BC) and submit himself to him, he must not necessarily expect to have his treatment explained: in the *Laws* (720) Plato outlines two forms of treatment, corresponding to two modes of legislation, the authoritarian and the persuasive (Jouanna 1978), and in the *Republic* (389b) rulers are the doctors of expert judgement who will know how to use the remedy (*pharmakon*) of lying. There is also the expectation that medical treatment will be painful: Plato does not refer specifically in a political context to surgery and cautery – 'the twin horrors of pre-anaesthetic surgery', as Dodds (1959: 210–11) calls them[6] – but references to them elsewhere in his works are common, particularly with the implication of necessary submission to a painful but beneficial process, and without being specific, *Laws* 684c, by stating that the patients of doctors and trainers are content if they achieve their results without great pain, provides an apologia for the use of force. The image of purging also occurs several times in Plato in a strikingly modern sense. In the *Politicus* the Eleatic Stranger suggests that true rulers may on their own authority carry out violent purges 'killing or else expelling individuals' (293d, cf. 308e–9a, where the same policies are discussed literally). In the *Laws* (735d–6a) the description of purges is superficially more moderate, distinguishing the gentler from the harsher, but even the milder option is essentially exile under a euphemistic screen. As noted earlier, whatever is good for the body politic as a whole can be justified, and the philosopher-statesman is the only individual in a position to make that judgement.

Contemporary political discourse in the fourth century seems to reflect the Platonic model, though inevitably in a debased form. We have already seen how the orators mimic Plato in offering a slightly richer medical language than that of the earlier period; they also want to be seen as doctors of the state. Demades (fr.64) claims that politicians, like doctors, should not be blamed for the disease, but thanked for their treatment, while Demosthenes, in an ironic variant, compares Aeschines' political wisdom after the event to the case of a doctor who fails to advise a sick man of the proper treatment while he is alive, but goes to the funeral and there specifies the régime which would have saved him (Dem. 18.243, reflected in Aeschin. 3.225). Medical imagery can also reflect competition between self-professed experts: Demosthenes likens the theoric distributions of his rivals to invalid food, which neither gives the patient strength nor permits him to expire (3.33; cf. *Pro.* 53.4), while Aeschines, accusing Demosthenes of divisiveness, contrasts his policy of opening new wounds (*helkopoiein*) with the amnesty of 403 (3.208). Like Plato, Demosthenes seeks authority for violent intervention, saying that Aristogeiton must be disposed of by cautery or surgery, like a cancer or ulcer (25.95, cf. 18.324 for expulsion of the 'incurable'). There is an increasing violence of language, too: Demosthenes called the Athenians *ekneneurismenoi* ('hamstrung') (3.31) and included among his imagery, according to Aeschines (3.166), the phrase 'the sinews of the demos have been cut away'; he also charged that the 'crop of traitors' had 'mutilated their fatherlands' (18.296), a slide from sickness to violent injury.

III

The medical imagery of the fourth century is, of course, shaped by personal interest, and usually wielded by men with an axe to grind. Plato, with his sense of intellectual and moral superiority, regards the whole of practical politics as in need of his expert treatment, while Demosthenes and his contemporaries wrangle in a squabble for access to the patient which Galen would have had no trouble in recognising. If, however, one goes back to an earlier and less self-interested discourse, the picture is, I believe, rather different.

One important difference is that earlier medical imagery displays little if any moral aspect. In this regard it is very different from the discourse which Sontag presents as associated with cancer in modern times. For Plato, of course, the practice of the statesman-doctor is tied up with the health of the soul and the moral good of the community, as emerges clearly from the discussion of punishment in the *Gorgias* (477e–9e), where it is the judge who is identified with the doctor. In the earliest medical imagery, although the wicked behaviour of their wealthy leaders is seen by the poets as having consequences for the whole community (Solon fr. 4.5f., esp. 17; Thgn. 39–52), they do not represent the sickness which falls on the city as a punishment of Athens or Megara at large. Indeed, the sickness of civil strife is never, I think, presented as sent by the gods, or as a judgement on the body suffering it, or as a reflection of general corruption. In that respect, this form of civic sickness is rather different from the plagues visited by angry gods on the Achaeans at Troy in the first book of the *Iliad* or on Oedipus' Thebes, which reflect fundamental problems in the health of the community on a religious or ethical level, and so naturally have a moral dimension; in the same way, the plagues and blights first threatened and then abjured by the Furies in Aeschylus' *Eumenides* embrace civil strife (861–3, 976–83), but only within the wider framework of their relationship with the city of Athens and its moral values.[7] The sickness of *stasis* is also always denoted by the neutral word *nosos* ('disease') rather than *loimos* ('plague'); the latter term embraces a complex of disasters which include failures of crops and of human and animal reproduction (Parker 1983: 257).[8]

In the earliest Greek literature there is certainly a perception that if rulers are wicked, the health and well-being of the whole community will suffer, while the city of a good king flourishes (Hom. *Il.* 16.384–92; Hes. *WD* 225–47; Hom. *Od.* 19.109–14). It would not be surprising if there remained in Greek minds in later periods a residual concern that the moral character of their leaders might carry risks for the city at large, as Parker argues (1983: 265–71), but it is far from clear that this carries implications of pollution or contagion, as Connor (1985: esp. 91–3) has argued, suggesting that there is an association between the demolition of the houses of those guilty of tyranny or treachery and the treatment of offences which clearly did attract pollution or divine vengeance, such as murder and temple robbery. While the process may well represent the same objective in both cases, namely the complete removal of the criminal and his *oikos* (household) from the city, the motives may well be different. Where pollution is at issue, it is obviously important to eject from the polis or destroy any trace of the perpetrator lest the polis come to harm through contagion: in the case of a traitor, however, it makes equally good sense to regard the razing of the house and ejection of the offender's body without burial as a retaliation against one who has betrayed the community by expunging that person and his *oikos* from that community (cf. Parker 1983: 45–7, 195–6, 206). Insofar as traitors and other political malefactors have made themselves subject to *agos* (divine retribution), this is the product of curses which the community itself has pronounced as a pre-emptive sanction to prevent such behaviour (Parker 1983: 193–6) and which they can hardly have believed would rebound on them. Furthermore, almost all the evidence suggestive of a belief that bad leaders could bring disaster on their cities through a form of pollution derives from the heated and self-serving context of later fourth-century Attic oratory (Parker 1983: 268–9), at a nadir in Athens' fortunes which fostered recrimination and personal attacks. As we have seen, for the politicians of the fourth century, medical imagery is associated with mutual charges of disloyalty, perceived as a disease in the body politic, or perhaps rather portrayed as such by speakers in order to seek a pretext for action by the demos against their rivals, an aspect more or less absent from the earlier imagery: only Herodotus perhaps applies medical language (*sathron*: 'unsound',

6.109.5) to disloyalty.[9] Where a city's leaders are, or turn, bad, there are purely pragmatic reasons for civic surgery, above all in the case of tyrants, who are unquestionably morally repugnant; yet even in this case, while it is true that tyrants are regularly presented as the worst disease which can befall a city (Pl. *Rep.* 544c; Aesch. *PV* 224; Isoc. 10.34, Plut. *Sol.* 29.5 (= Solon fr. 35W)), a city suffering from a tyrant does not seem to attract blame expressed in medical terms, and the same should apply *a fortiori* to references to other individual figures identified with disease such as Demosthenes' rival Aristogeiton, mentioned above.

One obvious objection to this view of sickness imagery would arise from the often perceived affinity between Thucydides' account of the Plague at Athens and his account of the *stasis* in Corcyra. Given that both seem to be presented as quasi-case histories, it has been suggested that he regarded the events in Corcyra as a kind of epidemic, and in both cases there are clear allusions to the collapse of moral standards (2.53, 3.82–3).[10] However, these allusions are concrete, part of the actual experience brought about by an epidemic in one instance and chronic civil strife in the other. The two instances are parallel and co-ordinate, witness the very similar treatment they receive, with a symptomatic description, indications that both accounts are intended to have a prognostic function (2.48.3, 3.82.2) and a recurrence of medical language in the introduction of his analysis of *stasis* in the Peloponnesian War; accordingly, the two are at most to be regarded as both symptoms of some sort of meta-disease, the wholesale collapse of civil society.[11] Moreover, Thucydides' reaction in both cases is direct (and disapproving): he regrets the abandonment of moral norms resulting from the disruption of society in both cases, but that reaction stands on its own, and is not extrapolated into any kind of all-embracing judgement.

This conclusion, if correct, may be aligned with another apparent difference, namely a much vaguer attitude to treatment, and a much gentler one. Agamemnon threatens to remedy any political malady which has developed in Argos during his absence by surgery: 'where anything is in need of healing remedies (*pharmaka*), we shall endeavour to turn to flight the harm of the disease by sage use either of knife or of cautery' (A. *Ag.* 848–50, tr. Fraenkel), but this threat is unique up to the end of the classical period (and placed in the mouth of a less than completely sympathetic character). Much more representative is Pindar's appeal to Arkesilas (*Pyth.* 4.271–2): 'You are a most seasonable healer, and healing Apollo (*Paian*) honours your glory. You must tend the ulcer's wound with the application of a gentle hand.' Reconciliation is the keynote of the poem, and it is natural to expect Apollo's support for a Pythian victor. A similar impression could be formed from the passage from Plutarch (*Sol.* 15.1) which constitutes Solon fr. 33aW (if indeed it preserves any of Solon's words): 'he did not apply any medical treatment or innovation (*kainontomian* – lit. 'new cutting'), afraid that he might throw the city into complete confusion and disorder and then be too weak to set it upright once more and organise it for the best.' Here the appreciation that treatment is itself traumatic engenders a cautious attitude rather than a radical one. In general, indeed, references to treatment are confined to vague mentions of *pharmakon* ('remedy') or *iasthai* ('to heal'), even when a specific measure is in view, as in Nicias' appeal to the *epistatēs* (presiding officer) in the Sicilian debate to re-open a debate already settled by vote and so 'act as physician (*iatros*) to the city when she has made a bad decision' (Thuc. 6.14).[12] Indeed, in the majority of references to the sickness of *stasis* in the sixth and fifth centuries, the figure of the doctor does not appear, and there is no specific allusion to treatment.[13] Nevertheless, I suggest that there *is* a specific medical significance to the image, and that it resides in the concept of the internal economy of the body as a balance between humours, and of the need to establish a proper balance between them.

This concept surfaces explicitly in political imagery in the late fifth century in the pages of Thucydides, when Alcibiades, perhaps as a riposte to the foray of Nicias into medical imagery just mentioned, speaks of 'the inferior, the ordinary and the really acute blended together (*xugkrathen*)' as being the strongest combination in the city (Thuc. 6.18.6); in 8.97.2 the historian himself observes of the government of the five thousand that it was 'a moderate blending (*xugkrasis*) of the interests of the few and the many'. Euripides, too, speaks of a blending (*sugkrasis*) of rich and poor (fr. 21, from the *Aeolus*). The inverse image, Alcmaeon's account of the internal economy of the body as an *isonomia* (equality of political rights) between the humours, permits us to trace the link between the two fields back to about the middle of the fifth century (Alcmaeon fr. 4DK; Ostwald 1969: 97–106). The later use of the image has been very well discussed by de Romilly (1976), who analyses the close link between ideas of balance and blending on the one hand and of organic unity on the other in early Hippocratic treatises such as *On the Nature of Man* and *On Ancient Medicine* and their application to political thought. What I want to suggest is that the basic principles behind such ideas can be applied to the image of sickness in the polis from its beginnings.

Of course, the application of the detailed concepts to political thought cannot antedate their articulation by the medical writers, but that does not necessarily preclude an intuitive appreciation of the organic unity of the body politic or of the need for balance and harmonious unity within it, and indeed such an appreciation of the value of blending and combination seems to be reflected in the use of words such as *mignumi* ('mix'; *LSJ* s.v. B.1a) and *amiktos* ('unmixed', hence 'unsociable, savage'; *LSJ* s.v. III.1a).

Such an interpretation would help to explain why the figure of the doctor plays a minor role in the early development of the image and (in contrast to the common later use of disease imagery as an interventionist's charter) the approach to treatment is much more cautious. Furthermore, the perspective from which disease in the polis is usually viewed is that of the community itself (or else of a non-expert observer looking at the community as a whole). From such a perspective, and considering the body politic holistically (and we have already noted the late and limited development of the hierarchical anatomical model of the body politic), the important task is to remedy the dysfunction in it with minimal harm to the body. How exactly this is to be done is not spelt out, but the implication is that radical measures are not likely to be favoured; better to leave the body to heal, encouraged by a suitable regimen. In fact, this is in line with the sort of treatment often implied by early Hippocratic writings for infectious diseases, in which interventions are cautious and relatively infrequent;[14] the only difference is that it seems to be implicit in the imagery that as often as not it will be the patient who knows what is best. A further attraction of the concept of mixture is that the optimal composition will vary from case to case or patient to patient, and indeed there is a degree of flexibility in the concept itself, which may be imagined sometimes as a tempering of a powerful element by a milder one (as in the dilution of wine with water in the symposium) and sometimes as the concoction of a recipe from a range of ingredients.

If this approach is correct, the fundamental concept behind the image of the sickness of the body politic is of dysfunction within an organic unity and of the need for this to be remedied; in its origins, however, it is the patient who occupies the central position, and the patient's interests, *as perceived by the patient*, which are paramount. Detailed diagnosis is also much less important than prognosis, and this, as Sontag (1979: 80) remarks 'is always, in principle, optimistic'. That does not make the image as a whole positive, of course – the possibility of a cure does not guarantee a cure in any particular case, and the patient may die, or remain a chronic invalid – but it is free from the authoritarian tone of much medical imagery.[15] In these terms, the sickness of civil strife is a problem and a misfortune, but not a sign of pollution or corruption, and to draw attention to the disease is to issue a rallying-cry for the highest form of community medicine.

NOTES

I am grateful to participants in the original conference at Exeter, two anonymous referees and Douglas Cairns for helpful criticism and advice.

1 Earliest examples: Solon 4.17; Thgn. 1133–4; commonplace: note the evidence of the lexicographers: Hesychius has *nosoun: stasiazon* (' "sick": in a state of civil war'), and Pollux 8.152 gives *nosein: epi tou thorubeisthai kai tarassesthai* (' "to be sick": used of states of disorder and disturbance'). Cf. Dem. 2.14 and 9.12: the commonplace used in the latter passage, *nosousi kai stasiazousi* ('sick and split by strife'), has clearly been inserted in full in the former by unthinking scribes, though two manuscripts have *stasiazousi* only (McQueen 1986: 140). Parody of a stock political trope: Ar. *Wasps* 650–1: 'It is a difficult task, and one calling for great wisdom ... to heal a chronic disease which has become inveterate in the city.'

2 Inflammation (*phlegmainō/phlegma*): Pl. *Rep.* 372e, cf. 564b; *Laws* 691e; swelling (*spargaō*): *Laws* 692a; fracture (*rhēgma*) and sprain (*stremma*): Dem. 2.21, cf. [Dem.] 11.14.

3 It should also be noted that Diodorus (11.50.4) cites the oracle in a quite different context, and to quite different effect.

4 Although Nestle (1927) argued that the fable of Menenius Agrippa in Livy (2.32, cf. D.H. 6.86) goes back to a Greek origin, the parallels which he cites (X. *Mem.* 2.3.18; Polyaen. 3.9.22; Aesop 130 [Perry]) do not concern the city, and the fable's purpose, to justify the Senate/stomach as sleeping partner, has no obvious parallel in the Greek world.

5 *arrōstia*: Hyp. 2 fr. 10, [D.] 11.14; *katabolē* … *astheneias*, *prosistasthai*: Pl. *Grg.* 519a; Pl. Com fr. 201KA [= Plut. *Mor.* 804a]; *sathros*: Hdt. 6.109.5; *hupoulos*: Pl. *Grg.* 518e; *eklelusthai*: Dem. 19.224. I exclude *paligkotōs* (Hdt. 4.156.1), *pace* How and Wells 1912: *ad loc.*, since *paligkot-* does not appear in any of the Hippocratic treatises commonly regarded as possibly datable to the fifth century. In later treatises (*Art.* 19, 27, 40, 67, 86(2), 87; *Epid.* 4.20; *Fract.* 11(4), 25, 31; *Loc. Hom.* 43.3; *Mul.* 2.171) the principal notion is of deterioration and malignancy (almost the modern 'complications'), though not gangrene, for which the term is *sphakelizein*.

6 See in general Welcker (1850), a reference I owe to Vivian Nutton.

7 Cf. Aesch. *Supp.* 625–709, esp. 679–87, where the Danaids' prayers invoking blessings on Argos reverse a previous threat of religious pollution.

8 This outlook is also in line with the more rational attitude taken by the Hippocratics to the aetiology of disease, especially epidemic disease (Longrigg 1993: 33–46); for the wider spectrum of popular belief NB Parker 1983: ch. 8.

9 The implication of Agamemnon's use of the image in Aeschylus (*Ag.* 846–50) is similar, but his attitude is an anomaly for the period (below).

10 Hornblower (1991: 480) with references to earlier discussion.

11 Medical language: Hornblower 1991: 480–1; Swain 1994; for *stasis* as a real disease see Jennifer Clarke Kosak, in this volume. NB also, most recently, Kallet 1999.

12 For further medical nuances in the 'Sicilian debate' see Jouanna 1980.

13 Besides passages already cited, note Hdt. 5.28, Eur. *HF* 34, 272–3, 542–3; Thuc. 2.53.1.

14 NB Welcker (1850: 215–17) for cautious attitudes to surgery and cautery in practice, as opposed to the freedom with which they are deployed as a rhetorical commonplace.

15 That disease could potentially be viewed in such a relatively neutral manner is surely reflected in the very wide use of *nosos* ('disease') and *nosein* ('to be ill') to refer to difficulties of all sorts and *iasthai* ('heal') of their remedies, often in cases where we would more readily think in terms of mechanical malfunction: *LSJ* s.v. *iatros* II, *iaomai* I.2, *nosos* II; for *noseō* NB Xen. *Vect.* 4.9. In the public sphere such language can be used of personal downfall (Pi. *Pyth.* 4.293; Ant. 2.13), legal disability due to illegitimacy (Eur. *Ion* 579, 591, fr. 141 (*Andromeda*)) and legal redress (*IG* I^2 154.14 = *IG* I^3 164.28; Pl. *Laws* 933c), as well as of troubles afflicting the state: Andoc. 2.9; Isoc. 4.114, 6.101, 12.99, 165.

4

POLIS NOSOUSA

Greek ideas about the city and disease in the fifth century BC

Jennifer Clarke Kosak

My purpose is to investigate some Greek views about the physical nature of the city as they were expressed in the fifth century BC. I wish to ask whether the Greeks in this period considered the city a place of refuge or a place of danger and to consider whether their ideas about the nature of the city changed in response to historical circumstances. I will try to answer this question by examining connections made by the Greeks between human suffering and the geographical entity that comprised a city, and, in particular, Greek ideas about the city and disease. Disease is a potentially valuable point of reference because it is frequently connected with urban centres. Mirko Grmek has argued that population growth and increasing urbanisation in the sixth and early fifth centuries led to a corresponding increase in the incidence of disease in Greece, an increase which he maintains lowered life expectancy rates (1991: 92, 98–9, 104). While scholars continue to refine our understanding of life expectancy rates in antiquity, there is universal agreement among demographers and historians that urban environments tend to encourage higher rates of disease than rural ones (see, for example, Corvisier 1985: 59–63). Furthermore, Grmek's argument that many diseases can flourish only under conditions of relatively high population density is not, to my knowledge, contradicted by other researchers. Grmek points out that by the second century, the decline in health and the resulting devastation of the population was noticed by writers such as Polybius (1991: 98). Within the larger framework of an investigation into Greek ideas about the physical nature of the polis, the two questions I wish to address are first, whether the Greeks themselves indicate an awareness of this up-swing in occurrences of disease over the course of the late sixth and fifth centuries, and second, whether they came to associate disease with the city, urban growth or urban structures. The answer to the first question is, as we shall see, rendered obscure by lack of evidence; answers to the second question are perhaps more easily found, though it will become clear that the notion of disease contemplated here includes what many twentieth-century thinkers would consider both metaphorical and actual.[1] By envisioning the city as a place that is subject to illness, the Greeks in the fifth century anticipate what becomes a standard image in the literature of the fourth century (cf., for example, Din. 1.110 and Arist. *Pol.* 1302b34–42): the city as a corporate entity, subject to the stresses, processes and dysfunctions of the human body (see Brock, Marshall, this volume). The frame of such a city is, I shall argue, marked out by its walls, within which dread disorders can arise. By the late fifth century, the city walls, intended to provide protection for the citizenry, come to be regarded as structures that can also preserve, encourage and even breed destruction.

The impact of the environment on human health and behaviour

Let us begin with those among our classical sources who confront the problem of disease most often, that is, the fifth- and early fourth-century medical writers represented in the Hippocratic Corpus: do they perceive a relationship between urban living, density of population and disease? The answer is a mixed one. Although they do discuss the geography of cities with an eye towards the health or disease of the population, nevertheless, they do not single out the city as a particularly unhealthy place as opposed to anywhere else. The doctors are convinced that environment plays an important role in maintaining health or causing disease, but there is no indication, as far as I can see, that they see the city as a more or less healthy environment than any other. So, for example, *Airs, Waters, Places* specifically directs advice to the travelling doctor who will be visiting different cities and discusses whether a city will be more or less healthy or unhealthy depending on its geographical location. The writer maintains that the cities will have different diseases depending on their orientation to the wind and sun, and on their water supply. In his opening remarks, moreover, he urges the doctor to be aware of both the general conditions of a given country and the conditions peculiar to a particular town within that country (1.2–5). The author praises cities facing east and subject to north and south winds; the populations in these cities are the healthiest, he maintains, but adds the qualification 'unless other disease prevents this' (5.4). The information remains at a generalising level: we are not given any specific examples of cities that fit these categories. In the second half of the treatise, the author moves to concentrate on conditions at the 'macro-level' as he describes the physical characteristics of whole countries and races. Certainly this author connected the situations of both countries and towns with disease. Yet while he directs his remarks at cities with the assumption that doctors will be working in cities,[2] he gives no indication that cities in general are unhealthy as opposed to, for example, the countryside. He simply does not address that question.

Other Hippocratic treatises dated to the fifth century that discuss geographical issues likewise do not distinguish the city as inconducive to health. So the discussion in *Regimen II* covers some of the same territory as that in *Airs, Waters, Places*. The author discusses positive and negative effects of different winds and notes that the effects of the wind may differ depending on the type of landscape through which it passes. It seems almost impossible to find a healthy place to live from the facts presented by the author of *Regimen* in his climatological chapters (2.37–8). For example, the north wind appears on the whole to be healthier than the south (2.37.4), because the north wind is not naturally warm and dry; by contrast, the warm, dry south wind extracts moisture from the earth, the sea and all living things in an attempt to counteract its natural dryness (2.38.3–4). However, the north wind is naturally cold and wet: if excessively so, it can cause illness.[3] Thus, the author maintains that mountain towns facing north are not healthy (2.37.4); yet neither are those that face south (2.37.3). Places deprived of the north wind are not healthy either, but islands out in the sea are better places in winter because they are not so affected by the cold coming in from the north. Any winds coming over the mountains provoke diseases, not only because they are dry, but also because they stir up the air which humans breathe (2.38.6). The author does argue that winds coming in directly from the sea or from cold, wet materials such as snow or rivers are healthy, but here too are qualifications: if the winds are too cold or if they blow over marshy areas, they cause disease (2.38.5).

Like the author of *Airs, Waters, Places*, the author of *Regimen* gives no specific examples of Greek towns or city-states when describing these different geographical situations. Only large-scale distinctions between Greece and other lands are mentioned. In fact, the author of *Regimen* confines himself to discussing only two peoples by name, the Libyans and the Pontics. Although the geographical information in *Regimen* differs from *Airs, Waters, Places* in some particulars, the text likewise makes no mention of 'the city' being more or less healthy than areas of lesser population density. Whole areas of terrain are subject to various conditions; city and countryside within the same area appear to share in these alike. Even when we turn to the *katastaseis* and case histories of the *Epidemics*, which are often specific to one particular city, no city/country distinction arises. Moreover, whereas the authors of *Airs, Waters, Places* and *Regimen* describe places which they deem to be most healthy, the authors of the *Epidemics* offer no advice on where to live. Perhaps this is not surprising, since studies have shown that these treatises are largely descriptive and prognostic in nature (see, for example, Langholf 1990). Although the *Epidemics* do give information about the weather and the seasons, little attention is paid to features of the landscape. Thus, while the author of *Epidemics IV* states that knowledge of both seasons and places is important to the doctor ('Constitutions, and what sort of things become greater and lesser in which seasons, places', [Smith]), he never gives any specifics about place, whereas he frequently includes information about the weather and the seasons. Perhaps there is an unspoken assumption that the reader will already know enough about the place if he is given a place-name; that is, given the information that the patient is in Perinthus, the reader can fill in the rest for himself from his own private store of knowledge. But it seems possible that the doctors were more interested in the weather, which is subject to change, and water, which also changes in response to the seasons and the weather, than in the particulars of the soil and the topography, which are constant features in the life of a given population.[4]

For the Hippocratic writers in general, disease results from the interaction between the individual, his or her nutritional intake, and his or her environment (see Nutton, this volume). With few exceptions, disease – at least the kind of disease a doctor might be able to treat – results from a process, a series of actions and interactions, not from invisible entities, the hands of the gods or *miasma*. Many individuals may respond to the same environmental conditions, but many individuals grouped together have no greater chance of becoming ill than a small group does. It is the constitution and behaviour of the individual and the impact of the environment that count, not the population density. The author of *Nature of Man* does discuss situations in which disease is affecting large groups of people and cannot therefore be derived from the behaviour and physiology of the individual alone: the disease, he explains, must be due to some *noserē apokrisis* ('sickly excretion') in the air breathed by all those affected and the solution is to breathe as little as possible and to perform a *metastasis*, a change of location (9). However, the concept of contagion notoriously does not play a role in Hippocratic thinking, although it was a concept available to them: the traditional form of religious pollution certainly involved the notion of contagion; and Thucydides mentions the problem posed by contagion in his description of the plague (2.51.5; see Longrigg, this volume). But the Hippocratics deliberately eschewed traditional religious conceptions of disease, and this may explain in part why they construct a view of disease that does not include a role for contagion (cf. Nutton 1981: esp. 1–16). Hence, while the evidence from the Hippocratic Corpus demonstrates a firm connection between health and climate, it does not help us very much when it comes to the question of the city and disease. None of the authors in the Corpus maintain that any one Greek state is healthier than any other. Nor is there any suggestion that high population density affects health. Now, as previously mentioned, the author of *Airs, Waters, Places* does suggest that there are some countries that are healthier than others: who would want to live in Phasis after hearing his description (15)? However, the political views of the author intervene to complicate his arguments from geography: thus, the healthiest place in the world to live is in Asia (12.2–6), but it does not produce the best men (16). The best, the most intelligent men of course live in Europe. The spirit and intelligence of the Europeans are due to the variety of the European climate (23–4).[5]

Both poor behaviour and geographical entities cause disease, in the Hippocratic view. The behaviour can become endemic and ultimately genetic, firmly linked to the terrain in which a given population lives. The interest in geography and its impact on behaviour is echoed in a number of fifth-century non-medical texts, most obviously in Herodotus. Like the medical writers, Herodotus generally emphasises large-scale distinctions between Greeks and non-Greeks, although he does intimate some differences among Greek states. This approach is no doubt in keeping with his overall story, which ultimately celebrates the free and independent spirit of the Greeks as against the slavish nature of the Persians. But other evidence from the classical period indicates that the Greeks did make more specific connections between the geographical situation of a given polis and the behaviour of its citizens. Thucydides, for example, emphasises the role that the relatively poor soil of Attica played in the development of the Athenian state (1.2.5–6). Several sources, although none actually surviving from the fifth century, speak of the thick air of Boeotia from which apparently derive both Boeotian stupidity and Boeotian appetites. Thus, for example, the Thebans have, according to Cicero, *crassum aer*, which results in bodies which are *pingues*: 'The Athenians have thin air, for which reason the residents of Attica are considered more clever, whereas the Thebans have fat air (*crassum*), and so the Thebans are sleek (*pingues*) and healthy,' (*de facto*, 7). While Thebans were known for their health, and for their healthy appetites (thus, the 'Boeotian pig' expression of Pindar, *Ol.* 6.90), they were also considered thick and unfeeling (*pachus* and *anaisthetos* are the terms used in Plutarch, *Moralia* 995e [*de esu carn.* 1.6]): there seems to be an association between the thickness of the air, the thickness of the bodies and the thickness of the feelings. Demosthenes also speaks of the '*anaisthetoi Thebaioi*' (*Coron.* 240). In *On Greek cities*, Heracleides the critic gives a long list of Boeotian defects, attributing a different defect to each Boeotian city (Thebes is known for hubris, fr. 1.25 Duke). But Strabo, refuting Posidonius in particular, denies the strong link between climate and intelligence; at 2.3.7, he argues that it is not by nature (*phusei*) that the Athenians are *philologoi*, while the Spartans and the Boeotians are not, but rather by character and training (*ethei* and *askesei*). The Athenian comic poet Pherecrates says simply: 'if you are wise, flee Boeotia' (fr. 171 Kassel-Austin).[6] Thus, although certainly contested, a link between the environment and human character, and thus to some extent human behaviour, persisted throughout antiquity. That many Greeks felt human physiology was influenced by the characteristics of a given city seems clear; whether they felt that specific types of diseases or increased incidents of diseases were brought on by city life or city topography is more difficult to discover.

The topography of pain: tragedy, the polis and human suffering

Tragedy is another body of literature where we find people suffering from diseases, although these diseases are often not easily defined in scientific terms.[7] In fr. 917 Nauck, Euripides explicitly refers to two important areas of discussion in Hippocratic medicine, regimen and environment:

> However many wish to practice healing well,
> Should when observing the diseases in the land,
> Examine the regimen of those inhabiting the polis.

Clement of Alexandria, to whom we owe the quotation of this fragment, cites Euripides here specifically in connection with Hippocratic views on the significance of environmental circumstances in the practice of medicine. Yet beyond a reference in Euripides *Medea* linking Athenian intelligence to the bright air of Athens (826–30), it is hard to find places in tragedy where geography and human experience are set into the same relationship as they are in the medical writers or the historians. However, many scholars have shown how tragedy does explore the large-scale differences between Greeks and barbarians that the medical writers and Herodotus discuss. Furthermore, some scholars have argued that the tragedians do connect certain types of behaviour with particular Greek cities. So, Froma Zeitlin (1990) has discussed the unusual nature of the city of Thebes, whose myths as they are explored in tragedy reveal the place as a kind of anti-Athens. As Zeitlin has shown, the tragedians suggest that certain types of destructive behaviour are endemic to Thebes. There are frequent references in the Theban plays of Euripides to the violent origins of the Theban people – they are descendants of the Sparti, the 'sown men' who sprouted up from the dragon's teeth planted in the Theban soil by Cadmus. The Sparti have an inauspicious start: once grown, they immediately attack one another until all but five are dead. If Theban rulers wish to lay claim to legitimacy, they must, it seems, be members of the Sparti clan. Euripides' stress on the Sparti and on the influence of Ares in Thebes suggest that the problems of the city are deeply embedded, ingrained perhaps in the soil itself in which the teeth were sown: from generation to generation, the descendants of the Sparti continue to fight among themselves for power and privilege in Thebes.

That the Theban myths which interested the Athenian tragedians do share many similar themes may indicate a real contemporary belief about the nature of the Theban environment itself – but we cannot be certain. As previously mentioned, Cicero contrasts the pure air of Athens and the thick air (*crassus aer*) of Thebes. Moreover, the stagnant waters of Lake Copais lie not far from land-locked Thebes. Greek medical writers would not consider thick air and stagnant water conducive to a healthy climate.[8] Beyond general references to the rivers Dirce and Ismenus and the famous seven gates of the walled city, tragedy appears to give short shrift to the notion that the geography of Thebes might influence the health or behaviour of its human population. But Zeitlin's work does show that certain types of behaviour are associated with Thebes, and her work has led me to wonder whether tragedy might consider the impact of urban structures that are not natural to the landscape; that is to say, are there features in an urban landscape not necessarily part of the natural geography but nevertheless essential to the topography of the city? And do these features perhaps affect the health of the population? For example, the feature of Thebes mentioned more often than any other in extant tragedy is the famous seven-gated wall. How does living behind city walls affect a people, as opposed to living a less sheltered existence?

In the next section of this chapter, I will explore Greek views about city walls in the classical period; in so doing, I am trying to understand how city walls were seen in terms of landscape: were they considered only a man-made construct with no geographic significance, or did they operate to some extent as a geographic feature like soil and water? That is, can city walls affect the behaviour and character of the citizens they surround, and do they contribute to the health or ill health of the citizenry?

City walls and political diseases

To begin, I wish to consider a particular topos recurring in a number of ancient sources which sets the physical city in opposition to the men that inhabit it. We begin with Alcaeus fr. 112 L–P, line 10, which reads: 'for men are the warlike tower of the city'; the supplement has been made on the strength of testimonium from Aelius Aristeides, who states that Alcaeus wrote: 'it is not stones nor wood nor the craft of craftsmen that are the city, but rather wherever there are men who know how to protect themselves, in that place also are walls and cities' (*Or.* 42.207). The idea that it is men who make the city is repeated in Thucydides 7.77.7, where Nicias, trying to encourage the desperate Athenians during the waning days of the Sicilian expedition, states 'for men are the city, and not walls or the empty ships of men'.[9] Anna Missiou has called attention to Andocides' focus on walls and ships in his speech *On the Peace* and shows how the orator uses the Spartan offer to let the Athenians have their walls and ships in such a way as to claim that under such terms the Athenians will maintain their identity and their prosperity. Although she does not use the evidence from Alcaeus and Thucydides just mentioned, she does argue that Andocides' interpretation of the terms of the peace treaty goes against the prevailing democratic ideology of the day: that is, Andocides may claim that walls and ships are elements essential to the identity of Athens as such, but this attempt to equate Athens with her physical features is, as Missiou argues, problematic and subversive (1992: 74–6, 174–6). The Athenians recognised the importance of walls and ships to their past successes in the Peloponnesian War: Pericles had urged the citizenry to abandon the land, come inside the walls of the city and rely on their navy for offensive warfare. But the history of Athenian war strategy also included the famous abandonment of the walls under the leadership of Themistocles. Athenian pride lay in their navy; they had a much more ambivalent attitude about the walls. Nicias in Thucydides must remind his listeners that neither walls nor ships are sufficient to the identity – or to the defence – of a city; his statement acknowledges the strategies of both Themistocles and Pericles but tries to undercut the importance of either strategy by focusing on the importance of the men who carry it out.

Finally, Aristotle, in the *Politics*, debates the definition of the city at some length. He suggests that part of the problem in defining a city lies in the Greek language, for the word polis can mean both the physical territory of the city (for which the word *astu* is also used) and the political entity of the city-state. He rejects the notion that walls are the determining factor in the definition of a unified city state (*Politics* 1276a25–27: 'Likewise, when should one think, when a group of people lives together in the same place, that a single city exists? Certainly one should not judge by the walls'), but goes on to insist that allegiance to a particular territory is an important factor in the overall definition of a polis.

Now, if one were to ask a Greek in the fifth century, 'how do you know when you are in a city?', what would he or she say? For an American living in the twentieth century, the answer to such a question might be, 'when I see a large number of buildings within a compact geographical area', or 'when I pass a sign announcing the city limits'. For most Greeks, I would suggest, being inside the city is synonymous with being inside the walls. Thus, in Plato's *Phaedrus*, Socrates and Phaedrus suggest that being outside the city walls is equivalent to being outside the city. Phaedrus explains that he is going to walk outside the city walls on the open roads, on the recommendation of the doctor Acumenus (227a), and Socrates, eager to hear what Phaedrus has to say about his conversation with Lysias, says that he will walk as far as the walls of Megara and back, a walk apparently recommended as a health measure by the regimen specialist Herodicus (227d3–5). A few sections later, when Socrates begins to wax lyrical about the beauties of the countryside, Phaedrus teases him for seeming more like a tourist than a native when outside the walls of the city, where, Phaedrus suggests, Socrates rarely goes. Socrates agrees, admitting that he is really a man of the city. It is not the nature of the wild that interests him, but the nature of men, and so he must be where men are (230c6–d2).[10]

City walls, including those of Troy and Babylon, Tiryns and Mycenae, Athens and the famous seven-gated walls of Thebes, are an important feature in the accounts of many cities in various works of literature. Indeed, evidence from both Herodotus and Aristophanes points to the significance of walls in the identification of cities as such. Thus, when Peisithaerus in Aristophanes' *Birds* explains how the birds can gain power over both humans and gods by constructing a city for themselves, he suggests the walls as the first structure to be built (551–2, cf. 837–8). Indeed, the walls are basic to the whole plan, for it is by means of the walls that the birds mark off their territory; by guarding the walls, they can intercept would-be intruders and prevent any attempts to circumvent their claim to power. Peisithaerus' scheme reveals the close connection between settlement and control in the Greek mind: he maintains it is the mobility and flightiness of the birds which has prevented them from gaining power before. Now, by building walls and setting themselves up as a polis, the birds will achieve power. Of course, along with their new-found centralisation and power come invasion, war and danger.

This relationship between settlement and achievement is also seen in Herodotus, most obviously in his section on the Scythians. He claims that the Scythians are very difficult to conquer in war because of their nomadic existence (4.46). The very fact that they do not live in fortified settlements is essential to the maintenance of their freedom. Herodotus' discussion of the Scythians thus acknowledges the danger of living in fortified towns: such structures become clear targets. Yet the lack of settlement is at the same time a mark of primitivism: city living, in Herodotus' view, is a key element in the development of civilisation. The mobility of the Scythians, like that of Aristophanes' birds, is feasible because they lack large fixed structures like walls. Yet that mobility prevents them from unified action and thus from achieving anything on a large scale.[11]

Cities that do not have walls occasion comment in our sources. The most famous Greek city without walls is Sparta. It is Sparta's example that we are urged to follow in Plato's *Laws*, where the Athenian Stranger argues that the ideal city should not have walls. Walls, he explains, afford too much protection and enfeeble the citizenry (778d–e).[12] Indeed, city walls, which exist to protect the citizenry, come to symbolise the weakness of the citizens they encircle. Inside the walls, the citizenry become embroiled in their own problems.[13]

The negative view of walls is also represented, I maintain, in Greek tragedy, especially in the late fifth century. The walls of Thebes and Troy are repeatedly mentioned by Euripides and less often by Sophocles and Aeschylus, yet the playwrights never mention the walls of Athens.[14] While the walls are meant to protect the inhabitants of these cities, they also seem to enclose and contain certain ways of behaving: they keep the foreign enemy out, but they also keep the domestic enemy within. The walls, emblematic of a city's strength and endurance, in fact hold the weakness of the city in their solid embrace. The focus on the walls of defeated Troy and chaotic Thebes underscores the doomed nature of those cities: the inhabitants cannot seem to escape the patterns of action that recur inside these fortifications. In the *Bacchae*, Pentheus refuses to accept the foreign Dionysus into the official cults of Thebes, while at the same time Dionysus drives the women to escape the repressive aura of the city: in Dionysiac madness, they rush out to the mountains to celebrate the god who cannot be contained by the shackles with which Pentheus binds him. Pentheus leaves the city to observe the behaviour of the women freed from the confines of Thebes only to be torn apart unrecognised by his mother and aunts and brought back into the city in pieces. Dionysus triumphs in Thebes; Cadmus and Harmonia are expelled, sent into exile. In the *Phoenissae*, the blind Oedipus is hidden deep within the city inside the house of the ruling family, a polluted individual whose curse has spread to his sons; the morally repugnant Eteocles rules within the city, the morally ambiguous Polyneices attacks from outside. The chorus of Phoenician women hasten behind the walls of Thebes in search of safety, yet the walls are not enough – walls require people to defend them and the defenders of Thebes are continually embroiled in terrible difficulties. Thebes is not sacked in the play, but this has less to do with her walls than with the self-sacrifice of Menoeceus, the *pharmakon soterias* (893), who leaps to his death from those very walls. Indeed, at the end of the play, hundreds of men have died, but the walls remain. Yet the audience who knows the words of Alcaeus knows that a city deprived of its people is not a city at all. Similar patterns of exclusion, of action played out inside and outside the city walls of Thebes, and of human destruction can be seen in *Antigone*, *Oedipus Tyrannus* and *Heracles Furens*.

The material substance of Troy is intertwined with the fate of its citizens to a remarkable degree. The chorus of *Troades* describe how the Trojans joyfully brought the deadly horse through the walls into the city, only to find themselves in the middle of the night at the mercy of the Greeks now inside the walls (515–50). Later they sing of Apollo who helped to build the walls, but who has now participated in their destruction (809–18). Poseidon appears at the beginning of the play, stating his role in the building of the walls (5–6) and explaining that he is now abandoning the fallen city, since deserted cities can do the gods no good (26–7). Hecuba, physically weak, is the city's most eloquent defender, but her verbal pleas are not able to save the city from utter destruction. With Hector and Priam dead and the women about to be led off into slavery, the fiery demise of the city at the end of *Troades* is an integral part of a play in which the women mourn for the walls and towers of Troy just as they mourn for Astyanax, the future bulwark of Troy, killed, thrown down from the walls by over-zealous Greeks. Troy is a place of doomed hopes, where Trojans are always destined to be defeated by Greeks, its structures destroyed, its peoples utterly routed. The walls of Thebes, however, remain throughout the generations, as the ruling families are destroyed within.

While walls are important symbols in plays set in Thebes and Troy, they are not an issue in those plays set in Athens – of course, I am only extrapolating from extant plays. But perhaps this is not surprising. As we have already seen, ancient sources reveal a complex attitude towards the role of walls in Athens. The Athenians were as interested in boundaries as any Greek, but their history, beginning with Solon who boasted of breaking down the boundaries of sixth-century Athens, shows a preoccupation with mental rather than physical boundaries. In the late sixth century Cleisthenes declared that all males living in the Attic demes, outside the city proper, were in fact citizens of Athens. In so doing, he expands the traditional institution of synoecism in Attica attributed to Theseus.[15] The Thucydidean Pericles makes very few references to walls or traditional fortifications as he persuades the citizens of Attica to move into the city, abandoning their crops to Spartan devastation. Instead, he focuses on Athenian sea power and suggests that the citizens think of themselves as islanders (1.143.5) – islands, after all, tend to be healthier, according to the author of *Regimen*. Moreover, it is the air of Athens, a thoroughly mobile substance, which is celebrated in song. As mentioned above, the *sophia* in which the Athenians prided themselves is linked with the bright air, which they breathe in Euripides' *Medea* (826–30). Thus, Athenian pride in their openness,[16] their *sophia*, their naval ability and with that their mobility, is reflected, I would argue, in the physical features of Athens which Euripides chooses to stress.

Cities which choose to rely on their walls, which are confined and confining, too conservative, too stationary – these are the cities which suffer dreadfully in Athenian tragedy; these are the cities which have chosen to emphasise place, property and boundaries more than is appropriate. I do not mean to suggest that themes of exclusion, inside/outside, boundaries and wholesale destruction do not appear in plays set in locations other than Thebes and Troy. Rather, I am arguing that the walls of these cities not only participate in the metaphors which help to tell their tragic tales, but that they also structure certain ways of thinking about these places, so that the myths which take place there could not take place without these physical features to structure them. Nor am I suggesting that Thebes in the fifth century was too concerned with her walls, such that the Athenian plays reflect contemporary historical reality in this regard, but only that the Athenian tragedians exploit the existence of walls in these cities to emphasise certain themes in their plays.

The *polis nosousa*

This investigation into potentially negative features of the urban landscape has shown at least two strands of thought in Greek fifth-century sources: one, represented in some writings of the Hippocratic Corpus, makes no strong distinction between town and country, despite its geographical concerns; the other, represented in Greek poetry and to some extent in historiography, does oppose the city to the wild, the inside to the outside, and often reveals the city as a place of struggle and suffering, a place where destructive patterns of behaviour may repeat themselves generation after generation. I have raised the question as to how the Greeks would have viewed city walls: as a geographical feature signifying the break between town and country, or as a man-made construct with no geographical significance.

Now, in an effort to bring these two strands together, I would like to travel down a final path, looking at places where the polis is explicitly described as suffering from disease. Our earliest extant references are in Herodotus, Euripides and Aristophanes. Herodotus describes Miletus as *nosēsasa ... stasi* ('having suffered from *stasis*', 5.28). In Aristophanes' *Wasps*, the son Bdelycleon apostrophises about the difficulty of 'healing an ancient disease (*iasasthai noson archaian*) inbred in the city' (650–1). While jury duty had been mentioned several times early in the play as the disease from which the father Philocleon suffered, in the speech of Bdelycleon, the disease inbred in the city seems to embrace a kind of submissive, almost slavish behaviour endemic among the free Athenians: Bdelycleon maintains that because of this disease, the Athenians are being cheated out of the wealth derived from the empire that is their due. This notion of an inbred disease is reiterated in Euripides' *Heracles Furens*. Euripides uses the image of the sick city extensively in the play: three times, he describes the land or city of Thebes as 'sick with *stasis*' (34, 272, 542); specifically, at 34 and 272, it is the polis that is sick; at 542, it is the *chthon*, the land. The first two usages may be interpreted as abstractions inasmuch as the word polis can mean both the physical city and the city-state; but the third usage clearly conveys a sense of physical disorder inasmuch as the word *chthon* has strong physical overtones.

Thus, beginning in the second half of the fifth century, we begin to hear the city in trouble explicitly described as a city suffering from disease, a *polis nosousa*. We can of course find disease imagery associated with the polis or at least political situations in earlier writers. Solon, Theognis and Aeschylus also portray problems in the city with images drawn from human physical experience. So Theognis writes that the city is pregnant, and that he fears what kind of man it will produce (39–40). The situation that he describes in the ensuing verses 41–52 certainly includes *stasis* and violence, but these are not presented specifically as diseases. In 429–37, however, he acknowledges a division between the activity of the human body and that of human society as he expresses the wish that the sons of Asclepius had the power 'to heal evil and the ruinous minds of men'. Solon speaks of the political turmoil in sixth-century Athens as an 'inescapable wound' on the whole city: he worries the situation will develop into slavery or *stasis* (3.17–19). Again, the corporal image of the wound does not evoke *stasis* explicitly, but the association is strong. Pindar, too, uses the image of the wounded city as he urges Arcesilaus to reconcile with the exiled Damophilus in *Pythian* IV. He addresses Arcesilaus as the *iatēr epikairotatos* ('the most timely healer', 270) and speaks of the need for a gentle hand in tending the pain of a wound (271). In the ensuing verses, he explains how easy it is to disrupt or shake the city, while restoring it is a hard task (272–4). Aeschylus likewise uses the image of the king as healer in the *Agamemnon*, as the returning king explains how he will handle any political difficulties arising from his long absence: if soothing drugs fail to have their effect, he will root out the problems in the city through cutting and burning (848–50).

Given the literary pedigree I have rehearsed, the imagery of sick cities used by authors in the late fifth century is perhaps not surprising. But the boldness of the imagery stands nevertheless. *Stasis* for Herodotus and Euripides is no longer just a problem that can be usefully described by the imagery of disease; it seems in fact to *be* a disease. By the time we get to Plato, the connection between *stasis* and disease is firmly established. Indeed, the notion of the polis as a kind of body subject to the diseases of the human psyche can be found frequently in both Plato and Aristotle. But it is the historian Thucydides who makes perhaps the most detailed study of the similarities between *stasis* and disease (see Rechenauer 1991: 320–6), although unlike his fifth-century counterparts, he does not ever use the explicit image of the sick city. Nevertheless, the connections between his portrait of Athens suffering under the plague and his narrative of the *stasis* at Corcyra have long been noticed. The *stasis* passage in Book III frequently echoes the plague passage in Book II, as it shows how *stasis*, like a plague, infects, corrupts and destroys the citizens (Rechenauer 1991: 340).[17]

To return to my original question, then, does an association between the city and disease develop along with the development of the polis in the Greek world? Thus far, the evidence presented has demonstrated that many Greeks used the notion of disease as a framework for describing the fact and experience of *stasis*. Did they really come to think of *stasis* as an actual disease, the kind of disease that Grmek is talking about in his discussion of palaeodemography and palaeopathology? To the extent that disease and *stasis* are both, for the Greeks of the classical period, a kind of discord, a destructive factionalism which results from a lack of harmony and common purpose in the body, whether of the polis or of the person – to that extent, we must allow that the Greeks may have seen *stasis* as a real disease.[18] But this statement to my mind opens up several more questions: if *stasis* is a disease, can a doctor heal it?[19] If *stasis* is a disease, is it caused by the same things that other diseases are? If *stasis* is a disease, is it connected with the cause that Grmek sees as responsible for the growth of other types of disease: that is to say, increasing population in the cities?

The fact that the Hippocratic Corpus contains no remedies for political *stasis* may give us our answer right away. Perhaps we should dismiss *stasis* from consideration. But the Hippocratic Corpus is only one source of evidence for Greek thinking about disease, a source which combines both very traditional Greek patterns of thought and more radical notions that try to overturn such traditional ways of thinking. So the idea of *stasis* as the essential city disease should not be set aside too quickly. The fact is that *stasis*, as analysed by our ancient sources, is caused by change, lack of balance among the various levels of society and instability. And of course, change and lack of balance are leading causes of disease, according to those same medical writers. Nevertheless, the shift from describing *stasis* as *like* as disease to *stasis* actually *being* a disease calls for further analysis. In his description of the *stasis* at Corcyra, Thucydides indicates that *stasis* in the late fifth century took on a violent character that was unprecedented. In his discussion, Thucydides does not suggest that such violence was something new to the phenomenon of *stasis* itself; instead, he argues that *stasis* is a part of human nature and human existence (just as disease is) and will be more or less violent depending on the human context in which it occurs (3.82.2). Thus, *stasis* arising in wartime conditions will inevitably have a harsher aspect. Moreover, for Thucydides, *stasis* is endemic to human populations. Nonetheless, for Thucydides, the *stasis* at Corcyra in 427 was the first of its kind in the Peloponnesian War and paradigmatic of what was to come later in the war. Of course, it is part of Thucydides' programme as an historiographer to show how the Peloponnesian conflict was greater than any that had preceded it, so perhaps we must consider his remarks on the extraordinary character of the *stasis* at Corcyra and thereafter with this aim in mind. However, if Thucydides believed that *stasis* was especially violent in the latter part of the fifth century, perhaps other Greeks did. Hence, if the phenomenon of *stasis* was perceived to have intensified, perhaps the language used to describe that phenomenon had to intensify as well, moving from the metaphor of disease to the designation of disease.

I would like to close with a look at how two late fifth-century authors, Thucydides and Euripides, bring together these strands of *stasis*, disease and the city. Euripides' *Heracles Furens* is a play that begins with a troubled political situation in Thebes: *stasis* has taken place in the city and an outsider, Lycus, taking advantage of the polis *stasei nousousa* (34, 272–3), has killed the king Creon together with his sons and has set himself up as tyrant. But political upheavals are not uncommon in the history of Thebes, as Amphitryon points out in the prologue: several generations of power struggles have preceded Lycus. These political problems in Thebes are emphasised throughout the first third of the play. When the hero Heracles finally returns home upon completion of his labours, he finds his family in dire straits, about to be killed by Lycus. The political situation is explained to him in some detail, and again the image of a disease is used to describe *stasis* (541–3). Heracles soon kills Lycus and perhaps a large number of Theban citizens. But directly after this occurs, he is driven mad at the instigation of his old nemesis the goddess Hera and kills his wife and children. However, the *stasis* problem so emphasised in the first part of the play vanishes from the scene. The play focuses instead on the personal tragedy of Heracles. At the end of the play, Heracles leaves the stage supported by his friend Theseus as the two set out for Athens where Heracles will be purified. Who will rule in Thebes now? We are never told. But what I wish to note is that this play is dominated by two diseases, the *stasis* infecting the city and the madness infecting Heracles. The *stasis* in the first part of the play is characterised by the notions of *nosos* and *taragmos*, sickness and disorder, and these very same words later characterise Heracles himself.[20] I would like to suggest that the *stasis* at Thebes acts very much like an environmental factor, an air of sickness and disorder, which infects Heracles when he arrives in the city. The madness is clearly sent by Hera, to be sure, but there is some suggestion in the play that Heracles has done a lot of killing even before he turns on his own family: he kills Lycus, certainly, but he threatens to kill a large number of the Thebans as well, and Amphitryon suggests later in the play that he has done so.[21] The death of large numbers of Theban citizens, the killing of children by their fathers – these are the images of *stasis* in historiography, too (e.g. Thucydides 3.81). Euripides is rarely monocausal in his approach to problems, and the emphasis that he places on *stasis* in this play is surely not accidental. Thus, it seems to me that two causal factors are at work in the demise of Heracles: the goddess Hera operates at the divine level, while the disease of *stasis*, a disease of human manufacture, affects Heracles' behaviour before he kills his wife and children. Thebes, as I suggested earlier, is a good breeding-ground for *stasis*: fighting among citizens is an integral part of its history. Heracles leaves Thebes at the end of the play, and Thebes, or what remains of it, is left to mourn.

Stasis is always a negative phenomenon in our literary sources, aptly called a disease because of its corrosive power. If explicit discussion of *stasis* vanishes from the *Heracles Furens*, this does not mean that Thebes has found peace. Rather, the play itself participates in the great changes and reversals that the characters suffer, and it changes its focus, proceeding not smoothly but through a series of surprises and disruptions. The play begins with a broad canvas, portraying the suffering of Thebes and of Heracles' family, but then focuses in to consider the sufferings of only one man. If divine forces are instrumental in causing Heracles' madness and suffering, human social institutions are in some way able to help him to live, if not to live happily. The question that remains unanswered is how human social institutions can cure problems that seem innate to the city environment. In *Heracles Furens*, *stasis* is cured by a trick of language and of dramaturgy: it is simply silenced. But the historical reality of *stasis* in the fifth century was not dispensed with so easily.

Finally, let us turn to Thucydides. Thucydides' narration of the plague of Athens states that the overcrowding of the city was a contributory factor in the harshness of the plague (2.52.1). Furthermore, the reaction of the people at Athens, who call Pericles' policy for the defence of Attica into question after the plague has struck, indicates that the Athenian populace may have associated the plague with the crowded conditions in the city (2.59.2). And Thucydides also notes that the plague struck the city of Athens and the 'most populated of other places' (*tōn allōn chōriōn poluanthrōpotata*, 2.54.5). Although Thucydides himself does not claim that the higher population *caused* the disease, both Diodorus Siculus (12.45.2) and Plutarch (*Pericles* 34) indicate a belief that overpopulation was a contributory cause, not just an aggravating factor. However, Plutarch and Diodorus hardly count as proper sources of evidence for the classical period in Greece: they may well have been influenced by theories of disease causation that were not current in the fifth century. Thucydides himself is rather coy in his remarks about the causes of the plague. In the description of the plague, he pointedly avoids ascribing a particular cause to the plague, but, as Paul Demont (1983) has pointed out, Thucydides not only mentions Egypt as the geographical source of the plague but also includes earlier in the history (1.23) other natural phenomena which precede the plague: earthquakes, drought and eclipses. Thus, Thucydides may be indicating an adherence to the belief that geography plays an important role in disease causation.

But there is one other nuance in those closely packed phrases of Thucydides that I would like to explore: Thucydides mentions that those coming into the city suffered the effects of the plague especially. He goes on to discuss their living conditions, in stifling huts during the hot season (2.52.1–2). Earlier at 2.17.1–3, he had described them living in accursed places, in sanctuaries and even in the towers along the walls and mentioned that the city simply could not hold 'them coming together'; 'later' they moved out along the long walls and into the Peiraeus.[22] This seems to indicate an easing of the overcrowded conditions, but it remains unclear when that 'later' is or what effect it actually had. For could it be that it is along the long walls and in the Peiraeus that they set up those stifling huts where they were to die? At any rate, I wish to note that Thucydides emphasises the difficult physical living conditions of the incomers. They are living in uncustomary or uncomfortable places, and thus they suffer even more than those who have established places to live. All these structures – walls, sanctuaries, houses, even huts – are manufactured by human beings in order to provide protection from animals, enemies and the elements, but in the case of the plague, they contribute to human suffering. The physical city of Athens, Thucydides asserts, cannot successfully hold the entire citizenry within her walls without severe consequences (I pass over the question of how many Attic citizens actually came in to the city, leaving their crops and houses behind). The city fails to protect the citizenry from destruction. Thucydides' description of the plague reveals the double nature of the city, a place which can serve as a source of strength in collective human achievement, but which can also serve as a focal point for the worst of human suffering and human error.

The evidence from Euripides and Thucydides, limited though it may be, does suggest that in the late fifth century BC, Athenian Greeks began to see the physical city as a dangerous place, where the disease of *stasis* found a breeding ground. The evidence from Thucydides also suggests that at least some Athenians associated overcrowding and confinement with disease (in the modern biological sense of the word). Whether this also means that they noticed a correlation between the growing population of cities and growing disease rates is very hard to say. It is also not clear that they associated *stasis* with overpopulation *per se*, though *stasis* was certainly a phenomenon of the city and therefore to be found only in concentrated population groups.[23] An examination of the history of *stasis* in the classical period does not show that this phenomenon – in all its varieties – occurred more frequently in the second half of the fifth century than in previous decades. In other words, *stasis* was not suddenly proliferating in the way that other diseases no doubt were, given the rise in population. Hence, the impulse to describe *stasis* as an actual disease during this period is not likely to be connected with an awareness that disease rates were rising due to larger populations (or any other causative factor). Instead, as I have suggested, it is not the amount but rather the character of the *stasis* experienced that seems to best account for the designation of *stasis* as a disease.

The evidence from the fifth century indicates that the Greeks believed that geography played an important role in the manufacture of disease and, moreover, that they began to consider the walls, features of the city landscape, as having an impact on human behaviour and thus on human health. Furthermore, they believed *stasis* to be a disease arising in the city – and indeed infecting the city itself, as a kind of corporate entity. The evidence that the Greeks of the fifth century noticed that disease was more common and that this was caused by increasing population is lacking, but they often saw the city as a dangerous, potentially unhealthy place, as the many strikingly dark images of the city in this period indicate. Our sources from this period do not reveal complete answers to the questions posed at the beginning of this paper, but they do indicate that as the Greeks struggled to explain problems, both political and medical, they implicated features of geography, population and city topography as potential causes of human suffering.

NOTES

1 If we try to limit our discussion to modern western scientific concepts of disease, we risk overlooking behaviours and processes that the Greeks themselves considered disease but that we do not. Hence, the paper will range over a wider array of material than might be anticipated in modern discussions of the history of medicine and disease, but it is hoped that this will enable us better to understand not only Greek concepts of disease, but also Greek ideas about the polis environment and its impact on human suffering.

2 As is suggested by his words at 1.3: 'Whenever someone arrives at a city with which he is unfamiliar'.

3 *Airs, Waters, Places* and *Regimen* disagree over the qualities of the north and south wind: in *AWP*, the north wind is cold and dry, the south wind, hot and wet, while in *Reg.*, as stated, the north wind is cold and wet and the south wind, hot and dry. On the correspondences and differences between the two texts, see the notice in Jouanna's commentary on *AWP*, 77–9.

4 López Férez (1992: 218 with n. 1) notes that many texts advise the reader of the importance of place in the scheme of human health, but offer little by way of specific diseases arising from a place itself. Meteorological phenomena such as winds and seasons are subject to much greater scrutiny and play a role in the development of particular diseases. Place instead tends to have an impact on human predispositions to certain types of physiology, disease and character.

5 The interaction between political views and scientific ones in *AWP* has been much discussed. Calame (1986: 97) stresses the subtlety of the Hippocratic account, arguing that it operates on a relativistic scale which he suggests reveals an 'ethnocentrisme mesuré'. As evidence for the complexity of the Greek view, he points out that the author uses the Ionian dialect and that Ionian Greeks live in Asia, the latter issue raised explicitly in Herodotus and not in the Hippocratic work.

6 For more on air and character, see Horace *Epistles* 2.1.244. Juvenal *Sat.* 10.50 mentions the *crassus aer* of Abdera. For sources and secondary literature, see Courtney's commentary on Juvenal *ad loc.* He also cites Menander's *Samia*, which mentions the *aer pachus* of the Black Sea region. The significance of thick air varies: in some cases, it seems detrimental to health, in others, it is beneficial. Thus, in *de architectura* 1.6 (24), Vituvius praises *lenis et crassus aer* as nourishing and healthful, in part because it does not move about (*propter immotam stabilitatem*); yet he is concerned about the air quality near marshes, where the stagnant waters send *graves et pestilentes umores* ('heavy and noxious humours') into the air. Cicero (*De divinatione* 1.129–30) quotes Heracleides of Pontus on the relationship between the dog star and health: if the star was rather obscure and the *caelum* 'concretum' and 'pingue', then the year would be sickly; if on the other hand, the star shone clearly in a sky which was 'tenue', then the year would be healthy. In this case, then, thin air is healthier. On the other hand, thick air in every case diminishes intelligence. Plato and Aristotle reflect similar beliefs about the connection between environment and intelligence: see Plato *Tim.* 24c4–d3; *Laws* V. 747d2–e2; Aristotle *Politics* VII.6. Later sources give fresh information: Megasthenes, quoted in Diodorus 2.36, remarks that the Indians are clever because they have pure (*katharos*) air and very fine (*leptos*) water. Vitruvius 6.1.9 notes that thinner air creates smarter people, although he maintains that stronger physiques are produced in climates with thicker air. Thus, southern climates (such as Italy) have smaller people of greater intelligence, whereas northern climates produce tall sturdy people of lesser intelligence *propter obstantiam aeris* ('because of the obstructive quality of the air').

7 Some of the material on tragedy in this chapter is drawn from my dissertation, *The Pain of the Living: Suffering and Healing in Euripidean Tragedy*, University of Michigan, 1994.

8 And, in fact, Boeotia would have been more prone than many parts of Greece to certain diseases such as malaria, because of the amount of marshy terrain present there. See arguments for this in Corvisier 1985: 10–22. Admittedly, he argues that Attica would have been a less healthy geographical location as well, due to its relatively flat nature and the marshy areas near Marathon.

9 On the extraordinary richness of the imagery used by Thucydides in this section, as he develops the idea that the Athenian troops have established a kind of city in Sicily and yet also act like a nomadic tribe, see Longo 1975.

10 'Phaed. "So neither do you go abroad out of the city to foreign territory, nor do you seem to me to go outside the walls at all." So. "Forgive me, best of men, for I am a lover of learning; and so while the countryside and the trees are likely to teach me nothing, men in the city are"'.

11 Compare also Thucydides' assessment of early Greek migration and settlement patterns in 1.2: he argues that many Greeks in the early period had no interest in agriculture or commerce in fixed locations, but instead moved around from one fertile territory to another, and power in fertile regions changed hands frequently; in such circumstances,

they failed to build any large cities or attain 'any form of greatness'. By contrast, Attica, not subject to invasion or takeover due to her poverty, managed to grow and prosper.

12 Note esp. 778e6–8 'if we should build an encircling wall, which in the first place is not at all helpful for cities with respect to health, and also usually causes a certain soft attitude in the souls of the inhabitants'.

13 Ducrey (1995) offers a diachronic approach to the issue of the importance of city walls in polis identity. He concludes that while city walls cannot be considered an essential part of city identity in the Dark or Archaic ages of Greece, they appear to have become by Aristotle's day 'sinon comme un élément constitutif de la cité grec de son temps, du moins un équipement indispensable' (255). He notes also a discrepancy in the classical period between the actual situation, in which many cities did not have walls, and the conceptual situation, in which Sparta is seen as the major exception to the general rule that successful cities do have walls (251–4).

14 The walls of Argos and Mycenae are also mentioned with some frequency, although it seems that it was really Mycenae that was famous for its 'Cyclopean walls'. However, Euripides frequently blends these two cities together within the same play. As Said (1993) notes, the tragedians in general represent Argos and Argive topography in ambiguous and changeable ways. Unlike Thebes, with its distinctive features consistently represented, the features of Argos/Mycenae are reworked and refigured with new significance in each play. Hence, it is difficult to discern a consistent pattern of meaning for the walls of these two cities as represented in different plays.

15 Cleisthenes builds upon foundations already laid down by Solon and Peisistratus, and also extends the important tradition of the institution of synoecism, attributed to Theseus (Thuc. 2.15).

16 Athenian 'openness' is further indicated in Greek tragedy by Athens' willingness to accept suppliants and polluted individuals within its borders; cf., e.g., *OC*, *Suppliants*, *Heraclidae*, *HF*. *Medea* shows that this tendency can be dangerous: Aegeus little knows the consequences of his oath to protect Medea.

17 That the Greeks were prone to see social processes as diseases is also confirmed by the recent study of Kallet (1999) on money as a pathological agent in Thucydides.

18 Rechenauer (1991: 341–51 and esp. 343) urges this point as part of his larger argument that Thucydides sees the Peloponnesian War in general both as a kind of disease and as a form of *stasis*, with *stasis* as a disease of the state.

19 Thucydides comes as close as any ancient author to such a suggestion as he sets up political leaders as doctors of the state. This model is particularly clear in the pair of speeches by Alcibiades and Nicias at 6.14–18, where both use medical language in their arguments over policy. See de Romilly 1976. See also Rechenauer (1991: 351–61) for broader arguments about political activity and its relationship to medical practice in Thucydides.

20 For *nosos* and the city see 33–4, 272–3, 541–3; for *nosos* and Heracles, see 1413. For *taragmos* and the city, see 532; for *taragmos* and Heracles, see 835–6, 907–9, 1091–3. Heracles himself will introduce *taragmos* to the city when he carries out punitive measures, according to Amphitryon at 604–5: 'Don't throw your city into confusion (*taraxēs*) before you set this matter right, child.'

21 Heracles suggests he will take vengeance on the perfidious citizens of Thebes who failed to protect his family at 568–73, but whether he carries out this threat after he kills Lycus remains somewhat ambiguous. But at 966–7, the messenger has Amphitryon refer to a plural group of corpses when he asks whether Heracles is being driven mad by recent slaughter: 'Surely the slaughter of the corpses (*nekrōn*) which you just recently killed is not somehow driving you mad?' See also 940 for another reference to the dead in the plural.

22 2.17.1–3: 'When they arrived at the city, for some few there was housing or refuge provided by friends or relatives, but many lived in deserted areas of the city and all the

sanctuaries and shrines except for the Acropolis and the Eleusinium and any other place that was securely closed. And many also made provision for themselves in the towers of the walls and wherever each was able. For the city was not able to hold them as they came together, but later on, dividing up the Long Walls and most of the Peiraeus they dwelt there.'

23 By the fourth century, Greeks were engaged in discussions about what size was best for a smoothly functioning city; perhaps these conversations were anticipated by Greeks of the fifth century who made connections between city size and violence.

5

DEATH AND EPIDEMIC DISEASE IN CLASSICAL ATHENS

James Longrigg

> The arrows rattled on the shoulders of the angry god when he moved and his coming was like the night. Then he sat down apart from the ships and let fly a shaft. Terrible was the twang of the silver bow. He attacked the mules first and the swift dogs, but then he loosed his piercing shafts upon the men themselves and shot them down and continually the pyres of the dead thickly burned. For nine days the missiles of the god ranged throughout the host.
>
> (*Iliad* 1.46ff.)

Here in the first book of the *Iliad* we have the earliest description in Greek literature of the impact of epidemic disease. The poet describes how Apollo, angered by Agamemnon's arrogant treatment of his priest, who had come to the Achaean camp to ransom his daughter, sent in punishment a plague upon the army investing Troy. At this time, Celsus says 'Diseases were attributed to the wrath of the gods' (*De medicina*, Proem, 4). Eventually, the Achaeans, at the suggestion of Achilles, consulted the soothsayer, Calchas, who revealed to them that Apollo had sent the disease to avenge his priest and that the god would not lift the pestilence until the girl had been returned to her father, without ransom and with a hecatomb of oxen for sacrifice. The Achaeans complied, cast the 'defilements' into the sea and sacrificed to Apollo. The god was placated and the plague abated.

A similar sequence of events appears in Sophocles' description of the plague at Thebes in his tragedy, *Oedipus Tyrannus* set in the mythical past. Plague has come upon the city. The oracle of Apollo at Delphi is consulted and it is revealed that the god is angered by blood-pollution. To discover the cause of this pollution the seer, Teiresias, is sent for. When it is revealed that Oedipus himself is the source of this pollution, he seeks to expiate it by blinding himself and going into exile.

Both these instances are typical in their superstitious reactions to epidemic disease. A god (here in each case, Apollo) is angered at some offence and sends disease. The cause of the god's anger is defined through augury. The god is finally placated and the sickness abates. It may be noted that the main concern in both accounts is to propitiate the god and eradicate religious pollution. Physical attempts to alleviate or eradicate the disease are minimal or non-existent. In the *Iliad* corpses are burned on funeral pyres and 'defilements' are cast into the sea. (The latter procedure may itself be part of a ritual of religious purification). In the *OT*, however, even this minimal sanitary requirement is neglected, and unburied corpses spread pollution.[1]

The Athenian plague by contrast was a well-attested historical event. It was recorded in harrowing detail by the contemporary historian, Thucydides, who himself fell victim to it. It occurred during the fifth century 'enlightenment' at a time when both medicine and history had felt the influence of Ionian rationalism. We might, then, confidently expect that totally different attitudes would have been displayed towards the impact of plague from the mythical accounts described above. But, it might be asked, would we be entirely justified in our expectations?

The Peloponnesian War broke out in 431 BC. In the early summer of the second year of the war the Peloponnesians again invaded Attica. A few days after this second incursion of the Lacedaimonian army, plague broke out in Athens – a pestilence, we are told, of unprecedented mortality. It raged ferociously during that year and the next, subsided, then broke out again in 427, wiping out, it would appear, about one third of the population of the city. The spread of the plague and its impact upon the besieged city is described by Thucydides in the second book of his *History of the Peloponnesian War* (47–54). Thucydides provides our only contemporary account of its depredations. No other unequivocal contemporary reference to the plague occurs elsewhere either in inscription or in literature. Thucydides apart, the first explicit reference to the plague occurs in Plato's *Symposium* (201D). It is curious that Aristophanes makes no mention of it in the catalogues of the ills of war itemised in the *Acharnians* performed in 425 BC. To explain this puzzle it has been suggested that the plague was too painful an episode for contemporary reference. (Thucydides' account would, presumably, not have been completed, or at any rate not have been circulated, until several years after the disease had run its course.)

Thucydides' rational, careful and detailed description of the symptoms of the disease is, for its time, rare – indeed, unparalleled, outside the writings of the Hippocratic corpus. Many scholars believe that the historian had been influenced not only in this particular respect but also in his general conception of history by contemporary medicine. Indeed, there seems to be no good reason to doubt that he was familiar with contemporary medical literature and influenced by the spirit of Hippocratic medicine. His whole methodology in writing history is influenced by the procedures of contemporary medicine (see Cochrane 1929: 16, 27; Weidauer 1954; Longrigg 1980: 211ff.; Rechenauer 1991). He sees human history as a 'great case book of social pathology' and seeks in his account of the Peloponnesian War to depict as accurately as possible the course, symptoms and the causes of that long malaise. His description of the symptoms of the plague epitomises both his general historiographical methodology and his historical purpose. His theme is the disintegration of Greek society. He is describing the processes by which social and political violence can undermine reason. The plague serves as a catalyst that expedites these processes. His harrowing description of the plague is itself dramatically exploited for historiographical purposes. The stark and immediate contrast between the optimism and confidence of Pericles' *Funeral Oration* and the grim ravages of the plague is deliberately heightened by their being set in close juxtaposition. By their very location Thucydides accentuates the deep-seated conviction that permeates his *History*, that there is an unpredictable principle, an incalculable element, inherent in human affairs. The plague is the unforeseen factor that undermines Periclean policy.

Thucydides records that the plague was believed to have originated in Ethiopia and spread from thence into Egypt and Libya and most of the Persian Empire (2.48). It then attacked Lemnos, then the population of the Piraeus, before spreading to the upper city. Although Thucydides refuses to speculate upon the origin and nature of its causes and leaves the matter to other writers 'with or without medical experience' (2.48), he manifestly does not attempt to account for the plague in terms of affronted deities as is apparent in the dismissive attitude he displays regarding the superstition that the occupation of the Pelargikon below the Acropolis would bring misfortune on Athens. Here he inverts the causality, maintaining that the occupation was not the cause but the result of misfortune (2.17.1–2). But, while he shares this rational outlook with the writers of treatises in the Hippocratic corpus, he does not also share the belief generally found there that epidemic disease is 'miasmatic' in origin, i.e. caused by air polluted by some unhealthy exhalation usually engendered by insalubrious weather conditions or insanitary location.[2] In his view the disease is communicable. It is interesting to note that Dodorus Siculus (*World History* 12.58), who clearly used Thucydides' description of the Athenian plague as the model for his own account, adopts a miasmatic explanation to account for its later resurgence and refers to heavy rains, stagnant pools which gave rise to putrid vapours, to bad food and the failure of the Etesian winds.[3] Thucydides himself, however, regards the disease, not as the general result of environmental conditions, but as individually contagious, transmitted from one victim to another by personal contact. He had observed that the doctors and those who nursed the sick were especially prone to catch the disease themselves (2.47.4, 2.51.5). He also records that, at the siege of Potidea, soldiers already investing the town and previously unaffected caught the disease from the reinforcements brought by Hagnon (2.58.2). In addition, at 2.51.6, he states that the recovery from an attack of the plague prevented (or, at any rate, reduced the severity of) further attacks (2.51.6). Thucydides has won praise for these observations and has been held to have been 'the first of extant writers to enunciate clearly the doctrine of contagion' (Crawfurd 1914: 37; cf. Poole and Holladay 1979: 295 n. 52) as well as understanding the phenomenon of acquired immunity (Poole and Holladay 1979: 299). But, although he certainly observed and recorded the *fact* of contagion, this is not to say that he anticipated the achievement of nineteenth-century biological science and clearly enunciated the *doctrine* of contagion or possessed 'an *understanding* of contagion and immunity' or had any conception at all of their true cause. *Observation* of the *phenomena* of contagion is very different from *comprehension* of it. And, in any case, by his own account, Thucydides reveals that he was not unique in recognising the phenomenon of contagion. He states explicitly that a number of his contemporaries were afraid to visit one another during the onset of the plague and that those whose sense of moral obligation transcended their fear and drove them to nurse their friends were especially vulnerable to the disease (2.51.5). Thus, although Thucydides may well have been the first to describe in writing specific immunity and the phenomenon of contagion, his own evidence reveals that the idea that one could contract the disease from someone already affected by it was a matter of general knowledge within the Athenian populace (see Solomon 1985: 121–2; Longrigg 1992: 34–5).

Another alleged cause of the plague is similarly implicitly rejected by him: that Peloponnesian sympathisers or spies had poisoned the water reservoirs in the Piraeus (2.48.2). Here we may discern a *topos* which, along with many others, is echoed again and again in descriptions of later epidemics, whose authors have taken Thucydides as their literary model, the view that epidemics were the consequence of plots by foreigners or external enemies. (We may recall, for example, that during the Black Death the Jews were accused of having corrupted the water supplies.)

In 430, as in the previous year, the Peloponnesians invaded Attica and laid waste to the country, whose inhabitants took refuge within the Long Walls. In consequence Athens became severely overcrowded. Thucydides himself mentions this overcrowding at 2.52, where he describes the refugees' plight in having to live in stifling cabins during the hot season of the year and camp in the sacred places. Aristophanes, too, with comic hyperbole speaks in the *Knights* (792ff.) of the refugees squatting in casks and birds' nests. Diodorus, notwithstanding his close use of Thucydides as his literary model, cites this overcrowding that had resulted in people living in cramped quarters and breathing polluted air as an original cause of the disease (*World History* 12.45.2). Plutarch, too, records that people claimed that the plague was caused by the crowding together of rustic multitudes in small dwellings and stifling barracks (*Pericles* 34.4). Although Thucydides here simply makes the point that the overcrowding heightened the sufferings of the stricken community, given his belief in the contagious nature of the plague, he must certainly have believed that it also facilitated the spread of the disease. Several modern scholars have found in the overcrowding described here clues to the identification of the disease. It has been argued, for example, that there must have been a consequent decline in personal and public hygiene creating ideal conditions for the spread of lice, whose infected faeces are responsible for the transmission of epidemic typhus, or for the black rat, which, when flea-infested, served as vectors for the spread of bubonic plague. However, it should also be borne in mind that the overcrowding might only have been for a time-span of months, at the most, and it is not certain that the period actually spent under these cramped conditions extended beyond the actual campaigning season. One might wonder whether what could possibly have been only a relatively short period of time would have been sufficient to bring about a radical decline in the Athenians' normal standards of cleanliness and sanitation.

We have seen that in the poets' descriptions of the heroic age few physical measures seem to have been adopted to counter the spread of epidemic disease. Let us now consider whether the situation was different in fifth-century Athens. Thucydides expressly records the failure and high mortality of the doctors when initially confronted by the disease. At 2.47 in a rather knotty piece of Greek, whose interpretation is controversial, he declares οὔτε γὰρ ἰατροὶ ἤρκουν τὸ πρῶτον θεραπεύοντες ἀγνοίᾳ. If the interpretation placed upon this passage by the scholiast ('if they had known that it was plague, they would not have attempted to treat it') is correct we should then have a fifth-century parallel to the cowardly behaviour attributed to doctors by the French physician Guy de Chauliac (see Nicaise 1980: 171) during the onset of bubonic plague in the Middle Ages – a view that has found some favour in modern scholarship (e.g. Lichtenthaeler 1979). This rather cynical interpretation seems to me preferable to the one more traditionally adopted, viz. 'the doctors at first were helpless in their treatment', since the latter implies that, although ineffective at first, this treatment later achieved success. But there is no suggestion elsewhere that the doctors were subsequently more successful in combating the disease. A third possibility seems to me the most persuasive, viz. the sick sought medical help in the first resort but, when they realised that neither medicine, nor any other human skill, could help, they then turned to the gods for aid.

Neither human nor divine aid proved effective, however. Thucydides grimly records the dead and dying lying one upon the other, half-dead people reeling about in the streets and around all the fountains in their desire for water, and the sacred places, too, becoming full of corpses. The Athenians buried their dead, each as best he could. Many through the lack of the necessary materials[4] resorted to shameful modes of burial: some hurled their dead upon another's pyre and set fire to it, others threw the corpse they were carrying on top of another that was already burning and departed. If we can trust Thucydides' account here it would appear that the Athenians at the height of the plague, at any rate, failed to implement effective civil measures for the public disposal of the dead. It does seem, however, that some steps were taken, albeit retroactively, to ensure a safer water supply in the Piraeus. At 2.52.2, the dying are described as reeling about the fountains in their desire for water and at 2.49.5 we are told that the sick actually plunged into the water-tanks driven by their unquenchable thirst. At 2.48.2 Thucydides had previously mentioned the rumour that the 'Peloponnesians' had poisoned the water-supply in the Piraeus. He implicitly rejects this story; yet it seems likely that either this war-time scare and/or the subsequent pollution of the water-supply, had convinced some, at least, of the necessity of making improvements to it. It may be noted that in his aside at 2.48.2 he remarks that there were not *yet* any wells there. Thus it may be inferred that, by the time Thucydides came to write his account of the plague, improvements to the water-supply in the Piraeus had been made. Some support for this inference may be found in a scholion on Aristophanes *Birds* 997, quoting Phrynichus' *Monotropos* (fr. 376K), that seems to imply that the astronomer Meton had constructed wells in the Piraeus before 414 BC. There is no ancient authority for this and the precise date for the improvement of the water-supply cannot unfortunately be determined. Archaeological evidence, however, suggests that water was led from the Ilissus to the Piraeus in classical times. So it would not be unreasonable to believe that it may have been the plague that motivated this enterprise. The rumour that the enemy had poisoned the water-supply together with the later pollution of the cisterns (2.49 and 52) would certainly have provided a strong incentive for the undertaking.

A more immediate physical response to the plague, however, is recorded in several of our ancient sources. In the early second century AD Plutarch tells us that the doctor Acron of Acragas, a contemporary and, as some believe, pupil of Empedocles, gained fame during the great plague of Athens by ordering fires to be kindled near the sick and so benefited many (*Isis and Osiris* 79, 383d).[5] This strategem subsequently became a not uncommon recourse throughout the later history of medicine.[6] Although Empedocles is elsewhere credited with certain feats of public health engineering, notably checking the harmful effects of the Etesian winds by stretching out skin-bags on hill-tops and headlands to catch them (Diogenes Laërtius 8.60 [D.K.31A1]) and curing an epidemic at Selinus by diverting a neighbouring river (Diogenes Laërtius 8.70 [D.K.31A1]), neither of these stories is credible[7] and it may be suspected that Acron is mentioned in the present context because Empedocles, who is elsewhere credited with this use of bonfires, was himself dead by the time of the outbreak of the plague. Galen, too, mentions the employment of bonfires to counter the Athenian plague but attributes its successful innovation to Hippocrates himself (*Theriac to Piso* 16 [14.281K]; cf. Pinault 1992: 35–60). However, it should be noticed that Thucydides makes no mention of either Acron or Hippocrates' association with the plague and specifically comments upon the failure of doctors generally to combat the disease. This silence, coupled with the late date of our sources, is strong evidence against the employment of such an attempted cure.

It appears, then, that with the exception of what appears to be a rather belated attempt to improve the water-supply of the Piraeus, few physical attempts of the kind familiar to us from mediaeval accounts of the plague were made to alleviate the spread of disease in classical Athens: no quarantine was imposed upon the stricken either in their homes or in lazarettos, there were no *cordons sanitaires* (fear was the only deterrent to visiting the sick); no health boards were established; there was no evacuation (apart, that is, from sheep and cattle that had been transferred to Euboea before the Peloponnesian invasion [2.14]); no attempts were made to purify the air and inadequate provision seems to have been made for the removal and disposal of corpses – at the height of the plague, at any rate.

As Hesiod pointed out often a whole city suffers for the sins of a bad man (*WD* 238–45). Despite Thucydides' claim that the plague was responsible for introducing a greater degree of lawlessness at Athens and that under stress of plague men began to live for pleasure restrained by no fear of the gods or law of man, there is ample evidence that many Athenians considered both themselves and their city polluted in the religious sense. Not only was the plague itself regarded as a visitation from heaven (Diodorus [*World History* 12.58.6]; Pausanias [1.3.4] and even Thucydides himself [2.64; see further below] provide evidence on this score), but it was believed to have brought in its train other religious pollutions. Under stress of the plague some ultimately became totally disillusioned with traditional religion, since it was thought to make no difference whether one worshipped the gods or not, since believer and non-believer perished alike. Others, in turning away from conventional religion, embraced orgiastic and ecstatic cults such as Baccanalianism, the worship of the Phrygian 'Mountain Mother', Cybele and that of her Thracian consort, Bendis and the mysteries of the Thraco-Phrygian deity Sabazius. In the last third of the fifth century Athens witnessed a widespread interest in foreign and ecstatic cults. Undoubtedly, the plague played an important contributory role in creating the conditions that fostered their proliferation.[8] Again, overcrowding had led to people camping in the temples and other sacred sites. When these unfortunates were stricken with the plague, they died there. Under normal circumstances holy places were kept clear of death, and even those who had recent contact with the dead were banned from these precincts. Now, Thucydides tells us (2.52), men had become so indifferent that refugees were not only allowed to take up residence in the temples, but were even allowed to die there, and having died, their corpses were either left where they lay or summarily disposed of without any regard for traditional burial rites. One might recall here how in the *Antigone* Creon's interdiction of the burial of the Seven against Thebes resulted in pollution of the city.

However, clearly not all Athenians lost their belief in traditional religion.

There is strong evidence to suggest that the impact of the plague heightened the more conventional religious sensitivities of others and thereby contributed to the development of a reactionary backlash amongst those more conservative-minded, who were manifestly most anxious to eradicate the causes of religious pollution and to avoid giving further offence to the gods. Having survived the horrors of the plague, some sought the aid of the healing-god, Asclepius, the son of Apollo. In 420 BC, during the Peace of Nicias, at the first opportunity, Asclepius, in the form of his sacred snake, was solemnly inducted into Athens and lodged at the house of Sophocles until a temple could be built for him (*IG* 2^2 4960).[9] Additional evidence of the strength of this desire to eradicate sources of religious pollution and to propitiate Apollo, in particular, may be seen in the Athenians' purification of Delos, his sacred island, in 426 BC by removing the dead and forbidding future births and deaths there (Thuc. 1.8; 3.104). Although Thucydides himself rather dismissively describes this operation as 'doubtless due to some oracle' (3.104), Diodorus is more expansive and explicitly links this act of piety with the plague, which, he informs us, the Athenians attributed to supernatural causation (*World History* 12.58.6). Thucydides also records that the Athenians revived the ancient festival of the Delian Games, which had been held in honour of Apollo and Artemis. Furthermore, we learn from Pausanias that Apollo was given the epithet 'Alexikakos' ('Averter of Evil') for having 'stayed the pestilence that afflicted the Athenians at the time of the Peloponnesian War' (1.3.4).[10] There is some evidence, too, of legal enactment to guard against further religious pollution. For the piously inclined, to offend the gods by denying or even questioning their existence, by replacing them by theories of natural causation, by criticising them for immorality, by taking up residence in their temples and sacred places, by failing to observe proper burial rites for the dead, or even by calling the sun, the apotheosis of Apollo, a red-hot stone, was risky enough in peace-time, but in time of war was tantamount to treason and giving aid to the enemy, since such impious behaviour would alienate the gods from one's cause. According to Plutarch (*Pericles* 32) a decree was passed which made 'those who do not acknowledge divine things or who give instruction about celestial phenomena' liable to indictment for impiety, and during the next thirty years many leading intellectuals at Athens were impeached in a series of heresy trials. This so-called decree of Diopeithes[11] seems to have originally been levelled at Anaxagoras with the specific aim of discrediting Pericles through his friendship with that philosopher. But even if the underlying motivation was political, the change clearly reflects popular opinion at the time. Clearly Anaxagoras would not have been impeached on grounds where popular support would not have been forthcoming. Our source seems to suggest *c.*432 as the date of the decree. Adcock (1927: 478; cf. also Gomme 1956: 187), has argued for the later date of 430 and has persuasively sought to connect it 'with the emotions evoked by the plague'. This later date seems to me to make better sense on both psychological and political grounds: the theologically more conservative, as has been seen, regarded the plague as a punishment sent by the gods and Thucydides himself observes that Pericles became very unpopular for a time largely because of the plague (2.64.1).

In conclusion, we may note that in the fifth century, as in the mythical accounts, there appear to have been few physical measures adopted to counter the impact of epidemic disease. In each case, by far the greatest concern seems to have been to eradicate sources of religious pollution and propitiate the gods, especially Apollo. It is true that Thucydides, demonstrably influenced by contemporary rational medicine and writing against this background of scientific enlightenment, himself eschews supernatural causation of disease. Yet one might doubt whether this attitude was entirely typical of his time. As we have seen, both Diodorus and Plutarch later record that the Athenians attributed the plague to supernatural causes and their attempts to appease Apollo are recorded by Thucydides himself. So, although we might have expected totally different attitudes in the fifth century in the light of the development of rational medicine, little or no practical innovations were introduced to counter epidemic disease.

NOTES

1 In the opening scene of *OT* (4) the stricken city is described as being full of the reek of incense which may have been burnt as a public health measure as well as an offering to the gods. Odysseus, it will be recalled, employed fire and sulphur to cleanse his ancestral hall after the slaughter of the suitors (*Od.* 22.481–2). While it is possible that some degree of physical cleansing as well as the eradication of religious pollution may have been implicit in this action, given the divine associations inherent in the Greek word for sulphur (*theeion*), there seems to be little doubt that it is the idea of religious cleansing that is paramount here. See, further, Russo et al. (1992) on 22.481.

2 See, for example, *Nature of Man* 9.44ff.: 'But whenever an epidemic of a single disease is prevalent, it is clear that the cause is not regimen but what we breathe and that this gives off some unhealthy exhalation', and *Breaths* 6.19ff.: 'so then whenever the air has been infected with such pollutions [*miasmasin*] as are hostile to the human race, then men fall sick.'

3 It is interesting to observe that Diodorus puts forward this miasmatic explanation for the resurgence of the plague, not for its original outbreak. Thucydides himself had declared that the year of the outbreak was particularly free from other kinds of disease, which would seem to entail that the weather was good at the time. Diodorus, it appears, although seemingly committed to a miasmatic explanation of the Athenian plague, was evidently unwilling to set himself in explicit opposition to Thucydides here. We may further note that in his account of the epidemic that afflicted the Carthaginians investing Syracuse in 397 BC (*World History* 14.70.4–71), similarly closely modelled upon Thucydides' description of the Athenian plague, he also resorts to miasmatic (as well as supernatural) causation.

4 The text here at 2.52.4 is ambiguous: *spanei tōn epitēdeiōn* could indicate either that they had insufficient help to organise a proper funeral because they had suffered numerous deaths of friends and/or relatives earlier, or that they were unable to do so because earlier deaths had resulted in a lack of suitable materials for the funeral pyre.

5 During the previous century Pliny had recorded that both Empedocles and Hippocrates had adopted this practice of lighting fires to alleviate epidemic disease (*Natural History* 36.69).

6 For evidence of its use as an attempt to counter the Black Death see, for example, Boghurst 1894: 62–3; and to counter cholera in England in the 1830s see Longmate 1966: 53; Morris 1976: 173.

7 The former story is suspiciously evocative of Aeolus' confining the winds in a bag (*Od.* 10.19ff.) and looks like an embellishment upon Empedocles' promise to Pausanias in fr. 111 that he will be able to 'arrest the violence of the weariless winds that arise to sweep the earth and waste the fields'. The latter story, previously believed to be confirmed by contemporary numismatic evidence, is also highly unlikely and may be dismissed on geographical grounds. See Longrigg 1994: 34–42.

8 The cult of Bendis was accorded state recognition at the Piraeus in 430/29 BC. The Adonia is first mentioned by Cratinus (fr. 17), who is spoken of as already dead in 421 by Aristophanes at *Peace* 700. Cybele is referred to at *Birds* 877 (414 BC) as is Sabazius, who is earlier mentioned at *Wasps* 9 (422 BC). Aristophanes, apparently, wrote a whole play, the *Horae*, about these foreign gods in which, according to Cicero (*De legibus* 2.37), 'Sabazius and certain other foreign gods were put on trial and sentenced to be banished from Athens'.

9 Shortly after the outbreak of the plague, the Athenians mounted an abortive expedition against several places in the Peloponnese including Epidaurus, the site of Asclepius' main sanctuary (Thuc. 2.56.4). Doubtless they had good strategic reasons for doing so. But, at the same time, it would be unwise in the light of subsequent events to discount religious motivation altogether and underestimate Athenian desire for access to the god of healing.

10 Pausanias here refers to the statue of Apollo Alexikakos in the Agora at Athens, which, he says, was made by Calamis. His evidence has been rejected by modern scholars on the grounds that Calamis' artistic activity seems to have belonged to the first half of the fifth century BC, but Pausanias does not actually state that the statue was 'set up on the occasion of this pestilence' (*pace* e.g. Gomme 1956: 160), only that it was believed that Apollo was given this epithet for having stayed the pestilence. It is possible that this epithet was subsequently associated with a statue of Apollo that actually pre-dated the outbreak of the plague.

11 As recorded here by Plutarch the decree has evidently undergone a certain amount of rewriting and its authenticity has been attacked on the grounds that Plutarch is our sole source and there is no reference to it in other authors who might have been expected to mention it had it been known to them. Dover (1975: 24–5) regards Plutarch's evidence at best as not more than a proposal made by Diopeithes 'on some occasion (e.g. the plague) ... and ... transmitted to posterity ... by reference in a speech'. Even this minimal acceptance is sufficient for my present purposes here.

6

MEDICAL THOUGHTS ON URBAN POLLUTION

Vivian Nutton

In AD 232 Alexander Severus and his troops were encamped near the Euphrates frontier in Northern Syria, where, so the Greek historian Herodian reports, all fell sick in the stifling air (*Histories* 6.6.2). The troops brought from Illyrium suffered especially badly and many died, being accustomed to moist cool air and to more substantial rations than were being issued to them. The army was compelled by disease to retreat to Antioch, where both emperor and men revived under the influence of the cool air and good water of the city.

A modern epidemiologist, called in to diagnose a mass outbreak of disease in a military encampment, would immediately suspect some form of transmissible disease, such as shigellosis or another type of bacillary dysentery. The notorious camp fever, typhus, would probably be excluded from first consideration, as it requires a cooler climate for its vectors, lice, to flourish (Kiple 1993: 606, 676–9, 1080–4). An explanation would then be forthcoming in terms of insanitary living conditions, of infected water, of some form of pollution. By contrast, Herodian, like ancient doctors in general, ascribes this medical disaster in an army camp, almost a small town in itself, to poor diet and the inability of the troops to adjust to a new climate and its hot, stifling air. The water of Antioch restores them, not because of its purity and freedom from parasites, but because it brings about a change in the general make-up of their bodies: wind and water together counteract the heat and thickening effect of the Syrian desert frontier.

Herodian's brief comments reveal the gulf that separates modern medical explanations and priorities from those of the ancients. He focuses on different aspects of disease, he has a different view of causation, and his emphasis on habituation stresses climate rather than vectors, germs, bacilli, viruses and the like. In common with almost all medical writers of antiquity, he explains illness on the model of an individual's interaction with the surrounding air; receptivity and resistance, strengthened or weakened by diet or lifestyle, are crucial in determining the response to bad air, however that may be defined or explained. On this schema the question why the air becomes bad is secondary; what is causing the pollution is of less importance than the knowledge that the air has become dangerous. What matters, above all, is the ability of the potential patient to repel any harmful changes (Leven 1993; Nutton 1999: 141–66). Once the body has become accustomed to an environment, and provided that it continues to enjoy an appropriate *diaita* (a word that for the Greeks encompassed the whole lifestyle, and was not confined to the intake of food and drink), it is unlikely to become diseased.

With such an explanatory bias, there might seem little place in medical discourse for questions of public health and of urban pollution. Indeed, our surviving medical sources say next to nothing about them, although, as we shall see, what little they do say is not without interest both in itself and as indicative of the relative impotence of ancient doctors to influence urban elites. Furthermore, when medical men do turn their attention to such questions, their explanations differ considerably from ours. Cornelius Celsus, in the first century AD noted that town-dwellers were likely to die sooner than those in the countryside, a fact he ascribed to the effects of urban living, poor diet and a new luxurious lifestyle (*On medicine* 1.2). Pliny the Elder likewise explained the new diseases in the Rome of his own day in terms of a boom in luxury (*Natural history* 26.1–3; cf. Seneca, *Letters to Lucilius* 15.15–30; Plutarch, *Table talk* 8.9). Galen a hundred years later was not surprised that the skinny, dry, sunburnt inhabitants of Alexandria were prone to skin diseases that were almost impossible to cure. They were exposed to the hot dry air, and their diet was appalling; they relied usually on saltfish, shellfish, pulses and lentils washed down with barley beer. They also ate snakes, the flesh of donkeys and camels, as well as dates that were either unripe or prone to rotting. Their favourite titbits, pistachio nuts, although tasty, had no nutritional value whatsoever. Their local wine was thinner and more watery than the hot climate might lead one to expect, and was far worse than even the roughest vino of an Italian taverna (Nutton 1993: 11–31). Although the merits of Nile water had been praised highly by a previous medical traveller to Egypt, Rufus of Ephesus, Galen was not impressed, but he acknowledged that the muddy water of the river was vastly improved by the ingenious ways in which the natives managed to strain and cool it.[1]

There are other similar observations scattered throughout ancient literature; the pallor of mineworkers is a commonplace from Lucretius onwards (*On the nature of things* 6.811–17; Lucan, *Civil war* 4.298), and one can point in Galen, surely one of the most acute of all ancient observers, to a neat proof of the unhealthiness of life in the big city (*On the properties of foodstuffs* 3.30: 6.722–3 K.). You have only, he argues, to compare the fat fish that can be caught in the sparkling Nar, one of the upper tributaries of the Tiber, with the scrawny and smelly offerings that are found in the river once it has received the foetid outpourings of the city of Rome. Indeed, the detrimental effect of the city on fish can be perceived a few miles out in the Tiber estuary. No wonder that fish in the Roman market are sold off cheap. The city might indeed have a wonderful water supply, with lots of fountains and aqueducts (although not as splendid as those of Pergamum), but it is an unhealthy place (Galen, *Commentary on Hippocrates' Epidemics* 6.4.10: 17B 159 K.; 4.19: 17B 182 K.). The sewers that carry away the scourings from toilets, restaurants and baths, and the filthy water in which clothes and blankets have been washed, indeed everything that requires cleansing in a megalopolis, declare by their stench their capacity to pollute (Galen, *On good and bad juices* 9: 6.795 K.). In another passage, *On the preservation of health* 1.11: 6.58 K., when discussing water quality, Galen notes how water becomes polluted once a sewer from a great city or a large army camp has poured into it, or has had rotting animals, fruit and vegetables, and excreta dumped in it. One of his teachers, Sabinus, in a passage preserved in Oribasius (*Medical collections* 9.17: CMG 6.1.2.17) compares the fresh air at dawn with that later in the day, when it has become altered by the smoke, the smells, the dust, and the other effusions, *apophorai*, and odours of the city. This medical vision of the stinking ancient city recalls the evocations of the Renaissance city conjured up by Carlo Cipolla (1979; 1992) and Pietro Camporesi (1989: 63–77) on the basis of similar later medical texts, and of Enlightenment Paris as described by Alain Corbin in his *The Foul and the Fragrant* (1986), whose original 1982 title is even more pertinent: *Le Miasme et la Jonquille*.

Corbin teaches us to view smell not so much as a consequence or a symbol of pollution but as a polluting entity in itself. A foul odour, whether personal or communal, is a very physical thing, changed by and changing air. Hence ancient medical writers see no difficulty in equating its powers with similar noxious effusions from pits, mineshafts, holes in the ground, stagnant pools, marshes, or even clinging sea mist.[2] Diogenes Laertius, describing Empedocles' cure of the plague of Selinus ascribes its cause to *dysodia*, a foul smell (*Lives of the philosophers* 8.70). Others, like the physician Athenaeus of Attaleia cited by Oribasius, graphically recount how the air receives the effusions from marshes and lagoons and like them becomes putrefied, close and malignant, particularly in summer (*Medical collections* 9.12.6; CMG 6.1.2, p. 13). Only the marshes in Egypt, according to Rufus of Ephesus, are not dangerous, for two reasons: as he has himself observed, their waters do not putrefy, since they do not become overheated in summer, and the Nile in its annual flood sweeps away the old water and replaces it with new. Rain too helps to clear out the many miasmata that are in the soil, and allows it to breath freely (Oribasius, *Medical collections* 5.3.6: CMG 6.1.1, p. 117 = Rufus, p. 298 Daremberg).

These comments on marshes and fens, on stagnant pools and slow-moving rivers, were standard among Greek and Roman doctors of all persuasions, and, indeed, among all writers (see Borca, in this volume). The list of authors assembled 170 years ago by K. F. H. Marx in his still valuable *Origines Contagii* (1824, 1826) demonstrates clearly how the same observations and explanations could be found in all types of literature. Vitruvius, for example, clearly relies on a medical source for his comments on the generally unhealthy nature of lagoons and marshes, even if he then adds his own qualification that the climate around Altinum, Ravenna and Aquileia was extremely good (*On architecture* 1.4). This he explains by the fact that the sea not only can come easily in and out of these coastal marshes but also brings in salt water, whereas marshes are generally unhealthy because the air has become poisoned by the breaths of marsh creatures. More often, however, it is atmospheric and climatic changes that are considered responsible for the miasmatic pollution.

This tradition of interpretation extends into Byzantine times and beyond. Thus Eustathius, discussing the plague that opens the Iliad, informs us that Homer had got his medicine right, for he was merely putting into metaphorical language the truths of medical science (*Commentary on Homer* 1.1.41). Apollo's arrows were, of course, the sun's rays, heating and helping to putrefy the hollow plain around Mount Ida, and hence poisoning the air with noxious effluvia drawn from the earth. Homer was right to note that animals were affected before humans, since animals are more susceptible to these atmospheric changes. No wonder too that, in turn, when the weather changed, and the sun became less hot, the plague ended. The truths of medicine and poetry are thus united.

But, given that some doctors were aware of the smells and fumes of the city, of the dangers of sewers and stagnant pools, what assistance and recommendations did they offer? Detailed practical advice is curiously lacking. Rufus of Ephesus describes an army method by which water can be improved by filtering it through pits lined with sweet, smooth clay, the sort used for making pots, which will remove some of the nastiness (pp. 298, 344 Daremberg = Oribasius, *Medical collections* 5.3.29; CMG 6.1.1, p. 120). Galen, commenting on Rome's aqueducts and also on Nile water, as above, knows of similar techniques for improving water quality. There also grew up a tradition whereby smell could be fought with smell. Plutarch in his essay on Isis and Osiris (383c–d) mentions how physicians used to burn bonfires to drive away pestilence, making especial use of fragrant woods such as juniper and pine. Pliny associates this procedure with Hippocrates, others with Empedocles or Acron of Acragas (*Natural history* 36.69). Galen added further refinements to the story; Hippocrates burnt sweet garlands and flowers, and the richest of sweet-scented unguents.[3] His formulation of this Hippocratic legend, and of the healing power of sweet smells, remained standard well into the nineteenth century, as Jody Rubin Pinault (1992) and Alain Corbin (1986) have shown. That Galen, or at least his colleagues in Rome, actually put such theories into practice is suggested by Herodian, who reports that in AD 188, on doctors' advice, Commodus withdrew from the plague-stricken city to Laurentum, where the redolent fragrance of laurels purified the noxious air (*Histories* 1.12). Those who remained behind in the city followed their doctors' advice to make constant use of perfumes, incense and aromatic herbs, whose sweet odours, once in their nostrils, would, so it was thought, keep the foul air from entering the body through them. Alas, as the historian reports, the plague ravaged almost unchecked; many died, both humans and the animals that lived with them. Clearly Galen, or his fellow doctors, had not the same success as their great Coan predecessor, who, so Varro claims, had saved whole cities from plague by his learning (*On agriculture* 1.4.5).

Varro's appeal to Hippocrates comes in a passage in which he warns of the unhealthy location of certain farms and buildings; these can be remedied, albeit at considerable expense, but it would be better to choose a good site in the first place. Vitruvius (*On architecture* 1.4) repeats the same advice, both for individual buildings and for military camps and even for cities and colonies, while Columella, too, warns the farmer not to site his farm near marshes or a public highway (*On agriculture* 1.5.6). In late antiquity Vegetius delivers the same message for locating an army camp, noting that staying too long in one place, especially in summer or autumn, is likely to lead to a poor water supply and the befouling of the air through the smell of the soldiers' own excrement. Best to break camp and move to another location (*Epitome* 3.2). All this, as is well known, is good solid Roman practical common sense, part of their technical hygienic achievement.

What is less well known is that the same tradition can be found in Greek sources, and arguably at an earlier date.[4] Greek authors record the same ideas and recommendations as Varro and Vitruvius, but, in all likelihood, they derive them independently of any direct Latin influence. Oribasius, writing in the fourth century AD, preserves in books 5 and 9 of his *Medical collections* extracts from authors of the first two centuries AD, who are clearly writing within an existing tradition of environmental medicine, akin to that on which Vitruvius in the first book of *On architecture* drew for at least part of his theory. Athenaeus of Attaleia, the earliest of Oribasius' authors, notes how in towns the movement of air is blocked by buildings; it becomes close and thick, befouled by exhalations and increasingly unhealthy. Allowing the air to move makes everything healthier; one has better digestion, better appetite, even better sensitivity.[5] Similar comments are found in fragments of Antyllus, a Greek doctor of the second or third century AD, and in Galen's (recently rediscovered) commentary on *Airs, waters and places* (Antyllus, in Oribasius, *Medical collections* 9.9 and 11: CMG 6.1.2, pp.11–12; Galen, in ibid., 9.10: CMG 6.1.2, pp. 11–12).

Most interesting of all is a long series of extracts from Sabinus, a Hippocratic writer and commentator of the second century AD, who not only talks about the healthiness or unhealthiness of places in general and about the advantages of a south-facing, sunlit house, but expatiates at some length upon the best way of planning a city (Oribasius, *Medical collections* 9.15–20: CMG 6.1.2, pp. 15–20). Sabinus' ideal city has straight roads, orientated north–south and east–west, without obstructions, and with clear straight roads leading into them from the suburbs. Gentle winds can thus sweep through the city almost unnoticed, clearing away the smoke and fumes, while the sun can reach every house, no matter what its orientation. By contrast, if the streets are narrow or winding, the winds are constantly causing turbulence as they meet obstructions and are forced to change direction. There is a veritable battle of the winds, and the poor pedestrian feels as if he is being tossed at sea. Instead of carrying fresh air throughout the city and driving the bad air out, the winds go where they can, spreading foul air as much as removing it. Similarly the sunlight never penetrates in some areas, so that any exhalation, *anathumiasis*, cannot be dispersed. The air becomes thick and hard to breathe. This, says Sabinus, is true for a city on a plain. One built on a hill, however, is much better off without straight streets, for the wind blows foul air straight up to the higher ground. With crooked streets, the higher ground is much better ventilated. There is a sociological point at issue here, clarified by a passage in Galen alluding to Pergamum (Oribasius, *Medical collections* 10: CMG 6.1.2, p. 11): it was the wealthier classes who lived 'up the hill', not in the crowded streets below. Sabinus' advice keeps their dwellings sweet-smelling, insulated, one might say, from the noxious odours of the lower town.

Sabinus, Antyllus, Galen, Rufus and Athenaeus are recognisably writing in the Hippocratic tradition of meteorological medicine. Galen's observations in part certainly come from his commentary on *Airs, waters and places*, and it is tempting to trace the source of this interest in town-planning back at least to that Hippocratic treatise, whose purpose is, after all, to instruct the travelling doctor how to tell at first glance from the situation of a town just what diseases are likely to be found there.[6]

But if there was this tradition of medical interest in town-planning and the healthiness of towns, we may be faced with a paradox; that our medical sources say remarkably little about it, a point that is still valid even if we allow for the vagaries of the process of transmission. To judge from the fragments so far published from Galen's commentary on *Airs, waters and places*, although it contains many striking individual observations, he is not concerned much with the problems of what we might term urban pollution. Rather, and this cannot be emphasised too strongly, Galen, Sabinus and the other authors so far mentioned are almost entirely concerned with the effects of one's natural environment on individual health. The long discussions on the merits of different waters, such as we find in both the medical and the paradoxographical writers of antiquity, are concerned with water in its natural state (Ginouvès et al. 1994). The pollutants, if one may use that word, are those that are already in the soil through which the water flows; or due to the effects of sun or sea.[7] Likewise the discussion of cities is cast in the form of a consideration of the effects of their particular site, whether north- or south-facing, exposed to wind or in a sheltered vale. References to the effects of a man-made environment are notably few. If one lives in a city on a bad site, one is liable to fall ill with certain diseases, and these are likely to differ from those in equally unhealthy cities but on a different type of site. One might imagine that the only response would be to imitate Asclepius and his followers who deliberately built their shrines in clean, airy, high places, and remove to a better location (Plutarch, *Roman questions* 286D; Vitruvius, *On architecture* 1.2.7). But that is to misunderstand the thrust of the Hippocratic meteorological tradition: widespread diseases are likely to have a common cause, but particular manifestations of illness are those of individuals. Hence, as Galen firmly stated it in his commentary on Hippocrates' *On the nature of man* (2.3: 15.118–19 K.), it is the duty of the doctor to prevent his individual patient from falling ill, even if exposed to a general, common cause of illness in bad air or bad water. Hence, if one knows what diseases are likely to occur, what potential environmental dangers are present, one can take precautions in advance by regulating one's individual lifestyle. Here is the role for the doctor, as adviser to the individual patient, not to any official body, and it is at the bedside or in a consultation that he can best keep his patient free from ills.

This attitude, that the duty of the doctor is to deal with the individual and not to become involved in what we might see as matters of public health, was not confined to doctors. One has only to glance at the formula for the appointment of a count of the *archiatri* in Cassiodorus which details the duties of an official doctor, a *comes archiatrorum*, in late antiquity, a far more ordered and regulated society than in Galen's day (*Varieties* 6.19). According to Cassiodorus, the doctor's role was entirely one of treating the individual patient. True, at times city or imperial officials made use of physicians for their own purposes, notably in commissioning reports on assaults and murders (e.g. P.Oslo 95–6; P.Oxy 51, 475, 2111, 2563, 3195; PSI 455; Stud. Pal. 1.8) but we are very far from the Enlightenment world of Johann Peter Frank and his *Medizinische Polizey* (1780, 1976), let alone that of medical officers of health and environmental inspectors. Despite familiar claims to the contrary, in George Rosen's *History of Public Health* (Rosen 1993: 6–26) or, most, recently in Ann Carmichael's survey for the *Cambridge World History of Human Disease* (Carmichael 1993: 192–200), there was little or no connection between the practitioners of ancient medicine and public health. The 42 pages and 228 footnotes of a survey article on Roman medicine and public health only serve to demonstrate the width of the gap between the perceptions of antiquity and our own (Scarborough 1981: cf. Jackson 1988: 32–55). Soap, like public lavatories, might result in a cleaner and more fragrant environment, but its provision, still less its use, was not the responsibility of doctors.

Besides, questions of public health, of sewers, aqueducts, the removal of market rubbish, plague control, quarantine and the like are questions of political and social control. A doctor's recommendation to send a sufferer from a contagious skin disease out to the desert, or to exclude (or even kill) the plague-stricken was impossible to put into action without effective force, at either a state or a local level.[8] Modern studies of plague control in Renaissance Italy have emphasised this point over and over again (Palmer 1978; Cipolla 1981; Slack 1985; Carmichael 1986). Even when the medical man advised, his advice required the assistance of political and economic elites to be put into practice. An ancient doctor was rarely in a position to influence, let alone join, those elites. Neither the travelling Hippocratic physician nor the Roman doctor enjoyed much social status, and while one might easily imagine a Galen or a Sabinus in Roman Asia Minor as a member of the local town council, their contemporaries in Roman Egypt we know to have been far humbler men (Nutton 1992: 15–58; Pleket 1995: 27–34). Even when a doctor served as a magistrate, or as an *astynomos* (market inspector), there is no reason to think that his expectations differed from those of his fellow officials. A passion for fountains, aqueducts, baths and even enclosed sewers was not confined to medics, and Galen's passing comments on those who practise banausic arts do not suggest a widespread sympathy or desire to ameliorate by public means the environment of the lower orders (*On the preservation of health* 1.12: 6.61 K.).

In short, there was urban pollution in antiquity, and some of its ill-effects were noted by ancient medical writers, who from time to time offered suggestions for reducing them. But they had no concept of what we might think of as public health; a healthy community was one made up of healthy individuals, and the doctor's concern was with those individuals, not with any larger entity, like the city state or the republic. Even if he had practical programmes in mind, he was rarely in any position to influence directly the implementation of policies or of relevant building projects. The status, importance and power of medicine and the medical professions in modern society are very different from those that obtained in antiquity; to imagine otherwise is to fall into one of the subtlest, as well as one of the commonest, traps in all medical history.

NOTES

1 Rufus of Ephesus, p. 298 Daremberg = Oribasius, *Medical collections* 5. 3.6: C(orpus) M(edicorum) G(raecorum) 6.1.1, p. 117; Galen, *On the properties of simples* 1.4: 9.389 K; cf. Athenaeus of Attaleia, cited by Oribasius, *Medical collections* 5.6.3: CMG 6.1.1, p. 121.

2 See Marx 1824; Winslow 1943: 66–74; Phillips 1982. Galen's major discussions are in his commentary on Hippocrates' *On the nature of man* 2.3–4: 15.118–22 K., and *On the differences between fevers* 1.4–6: 7.282–94 K.

3 Galen, *On theriac, for Piso* 16: 14.281 K. There are no longer grounds for doubting the authenticity of this treatise, which was written *c.*AD 207, see Nutton 1995; 1997: 133–52.

4 That the Greek tradition antedates the Roman is noted in passing by K. D. White (1970: 416–21). There is no evidence that these Greek authorities thought of Roman practice, and their general coherence suggests that they did not see themselves as innovators.

5 Oribasius, *Medical collections* 9.5 and 12: CMG 6.1.2, pp. 8, 12–14. Athenaeus' date remains controversial. He was influenced by Posidonius, and hence most recent scholars

put his main activity in the last third of the first century BC. The older view placed him in the second half of the first century, if not under Trajan. The earlier date would confirm a Greek rather than Latin source for these comments; the later would not exclude it.

6 For this treatise, which survives in Arabic, and in partial translations in Hebrew and Latin, see Ullmann 1977: 353–65; Wasserstein 1982; Strohmaier 1993: 157–64; and Jouanna 1996: 133–48.

7 Rufus, cited by Oribasius, *Medical collections* 5.3.9: CMG 6.1.1, p. 118, used the word *miasmata* to describe what is cleaned from the soil by showers.

8 Caelius Aurelianus, *Chronic diseases* 4.13; older editions read 'cludendum' ('exclude'), recent editors emend to 'caedendum' ('kill'), which would indeed be a remarkable piece of advice.

7

TOWNS AND MARSHES IN THE ANCIENT WORLD*

Federico Borca

Introduction

Literary evidence suggests that the ancient landscape was studded with marshes and swamps. As a result, there was a close connection and a constant confrontation between the cultural reality of the city and the natural reality of the marsh. On the one hand marshes were unhealthy places, a source of disease and ailments and unsuitable locations for settlements; but on the other hand many towns were found in – or close to – marshy areas. Such proximity could convey disadvantages and detriments, but sometimes also advantages and benefits. The aim of this chapter is to make a limited contribution towards the study of this connection and confrontation between town and marsh. Many cities developed in marshlands and some of the most significant examples are explored here. The intention is to approach and compare the theoretical criteria believed ideal when founding a town with the historical reality and practice. In what ways was the marsh, a place that symbolised disease, death, and decay, associated with settlement and civilisation?

In ancient Greece and Rome the idea of civilisation was linked with a neatly featured landscape, the most evident traits of which were permanent urban settlement and farming; these stood as alternative choices to nomadism and to a subsistence economy based on gathering, hunting and sheep-breeding. The urbanised and farmed landscape was perceived as aesthetically beautiful and culturally significant. Wild nature, on the contrary, was seen as a chaotic, uninhabitable milieu, aesthetically ugly because it was shapeless and confused. Therefore, fallow expanses – mountains, woods, deserts and swamps – ideally needed to remain at the edges of the humanised space.

The marsh biotope is an environment rich in lush vegetation and decomposing organic matter. Its insalubrity often renders it uninhabitable and always uncultivable, for the plough cannot furrow its muddy extent. Both Greeks and Romans perceived it as a liminal area, irretrievably other compared to the spaces shaped by man and culture. It was a no-man's land where earth and water were mixed and jumbled; where movement was slippery and unsafe; and where only beasts, barbarians and brigands could feel at ease (Traina 1986; Borca 1995a; 1996a; 1996d; 1996e; 1997a; 1997b). So how and why was this space sometimes occupied by civilised man?

Marshes: unhealthy places for settlement

From the Hippocratic treatises it is clear that a healthy site was a prior requirement in the foundation of an ancient city. The entire *Airs, Waters and Places* is dedicated to the study of natural milieux in respect of populating and settling urban sites. In the *Regimen* (2.37,38,48) the unwholesomeness or, more generally, the negative connotations of dampish and boggy regions are explored. Furthermore, the treatises *On Humours* (12) and *Internal Affections* (45.2) devote attention to town orientation as well as to diseases produced by the effluvia of mud and fens. The problem of harmful miasmata, which are present in the air, is dealt with also in *On the Nature of Man* (9). Plato is the heir of this Hippocratic tradition: in the *Gorgias* (451e) and the *Laws* (744a, 747d–e) he asserts that certain places are better suited for human presence than others and emphasises the importance of a healthy environment. Aristotle is also conscious of the same necessity when in his *Politics* (1330a–b) he explicitly affirms that salubrity is a major and essential quality of the ideal position of a town, and that the availability of healthy water and pure springs is equally indispensable (see Rykwert 1976: 41ff.).

In short, when erecting buildings or setting up cities one should avoid fens, since they generate noxious animals and pestilential vapours, which contaminate the atmosphere, bringing ailments and ruin to everything. Varro gives precise advice about the construction of villas, stating that precautions must be taken in the neighbourhood of swamps where certain minute creatures breed. These creatures cannot be seen by the eyes but float in the air and enter the body through the mouth and nose causing serious diseases (*Rust.* 1.12.2; see Hooper 1934). The marsh *pestilentia* cannot be overcome: thus one must dispose of the property at any cost or otherwise abandon it. The damage comes from creatures whose invisibility emphasises the treacherous and unpredictable nature of their action and also the environment which generates them.[1]

Columella again stresses the necessity of not erecting buildings close to stagnant waters. The marshland, especially in summer, gives off a baneful stench and sends forth insects armed with stings; moreover, some swimming and crawling pests, deprived of their winter moisture and infected with poison by the mud and decaying filth, escape from the bog and stir up hidden diseases, whose causes are even beyond the clear understanding of physicians. Finally, at every season of the year mould and dampness corrupt and ruin farm implements, equipment and produce (Columella 1.5.6). So according to Columella the marshland causes harm to men in three ways:

firstly through the effluvium of pestiferous vapours, secondly by the generation of noxious wildlife – mosquitoes, amphibians and snakes which, infected by the putrescent sludge, leave the swamp and inflict other areas – and thirdly by the dampness which damages and rots everything. Hidden diseases that science cannot investigate, invisible even to a physician's skilled eyes, take the place of Varro's minute creatures.

Towns in marshes

Some time before Columella, Vitruvius had also noted that when founding a town one ought to avoid the dangerous exhalations of swamps. First, it is necessary to choose the most healthy site which will be high and free from clouds and hoar frost, with a temperate rather than a hot or cold aspect. A marshy neighbourhood should be avoided because the morning breezes of the town, when mixed with the vapours rising from fens, expose the bodies of the inhabitants to the poisoned breaths of marsh animals, making the site pestilential (Vitr. 1.4.1; see Söllner 1913: 13; von Hesberg 1989; Borca 1997c). There is no doubt that to choose a boggy place is always the last possibility: only necessity can compel one to build a theatre on level or marshy ground and when laying the foundations of a temple a hard and solid soil is preferable to a soggy and swampish one (Vitr. 3.4.2, 5.3.3). Nevertheless, Vitruvius adds that in such cases one may resort to the alder: 'frequently alder stakes, being fixed in marshy ground below the foundations of buildings, admit fluid because they have less quantity of it in their substance. Hence they remain imperishable to eternity, uphold immense weights of walling, and preserve them without decaying' (Vitr. 2.9.10: trans. Granger 1962; cf. Columella 3.13.8). Vitruvius continues to explain that Ravenna provides a good example since all works both public and private have such alder stakes under their foundations.

Strabo too mentions the architectural characteristics of Ravenna, the largest city in the marshes of northern Italy: it is a city 'built entirely of wood and coursed by rivers, and is provided with thoroughfares by means of bridges and ferries' (Strabo 5.1.7; trans. H. L. Jones 1923). This description is reminiscent of the marsh-dwelling community identified in the earlier *Airs, Waters and Places*, which explores the inhabitants of Phasis, the river of Colchis which rises in the Caucasus Mountains and flows into the Black Sea. The author specifies, among other things, that 'the inhabitants live in the marshes, and their dwellings are of wood and reeds, built in the water. They make little use of walking in the city and the market, but sail up and down in dug-outs made from a single log, for channels are numerous' (Hippoc. *Aer.* 15; trans. W. H. S. Jones 1923 [with modifications]; see Müller 1972: 138f.). Later in this passage, however, the author presents the inhabitants of Phasis in a negative fashion. In the seventh chapter of the work, the stagnant and marshy waters are analysed and deemed unwholesome and unsuitable for use. The dwellers of Phasis, a fen ethnic group whose physique and customs are moulded by an insalubrious natural environment, have bloated and weak bodies and are unable to endure physical effort. On the contrary, Strabo's attitude towards Ravenna is completely positive: he praises the settlement. Here the drift of the tide together with the river currents purify the swamps by removing their ooze and filth: hence human settlement becomes possible in a space usually populated by insects, frogs and snakes, and a flourishing economy develops, mainly based on controlling trade and inland waterways. The place is considered so healthy that it is chosen for feeding and training gladiators. Strabo concludes 'Now this is indeed one of the marvellous things at Ravenna – I mean the fact that the air in a marsh is harmless' (Strabo 5.1.7: trans. Jones 1923; see Traina 1988: 94f.; Borca 1996b: 125ff.).

So sometimes marshy areas could be regarded as healthy. The position of Ravenna was certainly not unique since many towns were founded in such circumstances. Strabo, for example, suggests a parallel with Altinum (a town in Venetia): 'Altinum too is in a marsh [*en helei*], for the position it occupies is similar to that of Ravenna.' The concentration of maritime villas on the littoral of Altinum, attested by Martial (4.25), indicates that the area reached a settling optimum, where convenient ways of communication as well as hunting, fishing and farming resources were combined with the salubrity and amenity of the place. Strabo goes on to inform us that the same phenomenon as at Ravenna is found elsewhere. In Egypt, Alexandria is the only city to develop at a site suited by nature for both terrestrial and marine trade, on account of the excellent port facilities, the canal system and the Nile. In addition, Alexandria had a healthy climate. Strabo explains that other cities situated on lakes may have heavy and stifling air in the heat of summer, because the lakes become marshy along their edges due to the evaporation caused by the sun. This results in an unhealthy air which can create pestilential diseases. By contrast at Alexandria, at the beginning of summer, the Nile is full and also fills the lake leaving no marshy matter to infect the rising air. Simultaneously the Etesian winds blow from the north allowing the Alexandrians to pass their time most pleasantly (Strabo 5.1.7, 17.1.7–10, 13: see Jones 1932; Borca 1998). Indeed Ravenna, as well as Alexandria, represents a miracle: the heavy fen atmosphere, usually dense with pernicious vapours and organisms, appears unexpectedly pure and salutary. Living or running water miraculously takes the place of dead and unmoving water and cancels out the *pestilentia* characteristic of boggy grounds. The analogy between these two cities then extends to the strategic level: if, in the midst of the marshes, Ravenna is unassailable, according to Flavius Josephus (*BJ* 2.16.4), Alexandria 'is protected on all sides by trackless deserts or seas without ports or by rivers or fens'.

Despite the idealised advice of some authors, marshes were not automatically bad. Fens were not all alike, and Vitruvius, although he cautioned against establishing towns in marshes (see above), was well aware of this. It is reasonable for city walls to be laid out in marshes, Vitruvius argues, if these marshes are along the sea, they face towards the north, or between the north and east, and if they are higher than the sea-coast. For if dykes are cut, when the sea is swollen by storms, it overflows into these marshes and the sea salt prevents the birth of various kinds of marsh creatures; and even if any creatures swim down to the coast, they are killed by the unfamiliar saltiness. Vitruvius cites as an example the Gallic marshes which are round Altinum, Ravenna and Aquileia; towns which have an incredible salubrity. Therefore, three essential conditions lie at the basis of the climatic suitability and the engineering rationality of certain marsh towns: the nearness of the sea, an altitude higher than that of the coastline, and finally the particular location. Of course, besides these favourable characteristics, which are predisposed by nature, there is human intervention. This permits, by cutting canals, the change of water and, consequently, the recovery of otherwise uninhabitable lands. Altinum, Ravenna, Aquileia and other *municipia* with similar topographical features are immune from malaria and swamp *pestilentia* because they benefit from a special and delicate natural balance, which can also be achieved by means of land-reclamation works (see Strazzulla 1989). By contrast Vitruvius notes that places which have stagnant marshes, and lack free-flowing outlets such as rivers and dykes, like the Pomptine marshes, become foul and give off a heavy and pestilent moisture (Vitr. 1.4.11–12; cf. Fedeli 1990: 105). Indeed, despite repeated attempts, the Pomptine marshes were never completely drained in antiquity (Hughes 1994: 107, 144).

Vitruvius continues by describing an emblematic occurrence of such an ecological situation, a real historical *exemplum*. In Apulia, the town of Old Salpia was situated in such a place and the inhabitants suffered every year from various ailments. Eventually they sought advice from M. Hostilius and made a public request that he should seek out and choose a fit site for the relocation of their walls. So he obtained a site in a healthy place, and gained permission from the senate and Roman people to remove the town. After establishing the walls, he opened the lake into the sea, and made a harbour for the municipality. And so, Vitruvius concludes, the people of Salpia now dwell on a healthy site. In fact the site appears to have remained so until the sixteenth century when the expansion of the marshy area forced its abandonment (Vitr. 1.4.12: see Granger 1962; for the *Salapina* or *Salpina palus* note also Lucan 5.377; Vib. Seq. *Geogr.* 5.11 [p. 68 Parroni]; for the *Salapinorum pestilentia* Cic. *Leg. agr.* 2.27; on Salpia see Gabba 1983).

The co-existence of marsh and town

The city and the marsh, poles apart in the ideal ancient landscape, could nevertheless coexist in practice, and sometimes even with considerable benefits for the inhabitants. We are informed by both literary and archaeological evidence of many cases. In addition to the urban settlements on the northern Adriatic coast, we can note the numerous towns which developed just behind the belt of lagoons and salt marshes in Gallia Narbonensis, exploiting the resources and routes of communication offered by those waters (Borca 1996c). In the interior of the province Toulouse and Vienne were founded in regions which abounded in watercourses and swampish grounds. Arles and Narbonne, situated in broad marshlands and lagoons, shared wholesome sites with advantageous positions for trade. In the late imperial age Arles was defined by Ausonius as 'the little Rome of Gaul' which collected wares from the whole Roman world and, rather than keeping them for itself, enriched the other towns of the region. Narbonne was hyperbolically depicted as a landing place for every merchandise from all over the world (Auson. *Urb.* 10.1–8, 19.20–1). A century later, Sidonius celebrated the healthiness of Narbo, the town and country both gladdening the eye alike; he lists every component canonical to the panegyrics of cities: walls and gates, porticoes, forum, theatre, shrines, capitol, baths, arches, granaries, markets, fountains, meadows and finally the harbour (Sid. Apoll. *Carm.* 23.37–44).

In Italy, the Po Valley was, for example, strewn with bogs (Strabo 5.1.5,11; Borca 1997d). In the region of Venetia, Padua was located in the midst of the marshland which spread between the Euganei Hills and the Adriatic sea; the ancients connected the name Patavium with a marsh (*Patina* or *Patena palus*), which would appear to have extended in proximity to the town (Strabo 5.1.7; Servius *ad Aen.* 1.274; Schol. Verg. Veron. *Aen.* 1.247). In Liguria, Vada Sabatia, so named after the marshes (*vada*), was placed in a barely accessible position: it rose between the Alps and the Apennines, in a boggy – even if fertile – plain (Cic. *Fam.* 11.13.2; Strabo 4.6.1). Marshes also stretched over the neighbourhood of Forum Gallorum, a village midway between Mutina and Bologna where, in April 43 BC, the soldiers of Antonius fought against the troops of Irtius and Pansa (Cic. *Fam.* 10.30.2; App. *B Civ.* 3.66 and 70; at that time woods and marshlands extended on both sides of the *via Aemilia*: cf. Frontin. *Str.* 2.5.39).

Marshlands, together with woods, were also characteristic of the natural environment of the site of Rome itself (Borca 1995b). There were also fens near Ostia (Livy 1.33.9; *CIL* XIV, 4285). Nero commanded the rubble resulting from the fire of Rome to be thrown into the Ostian marshes; this report, given by Tacitus (*Ann.* 15.43.3), points to a conception of the marsh as a dump. Afterwards, when the emperor Vespasian charged Lucius Vestinus with the task of rebuilding the Capitol, the consulted haruspices recommended that the debris of the old building should be cast away into a fen and that the new temple should be erected on the foundations of the former one (Tac. *Hist.* 4.53.2).

It seems that once even the Pomptine marshes were populated by twenty-four towns (Pliny *NH* 3.59). In this area we know of Tarracina, which was described by Livy as a city sloping down towards the fens and was abandoned, according to Pliny the Elder, because of the enormous amount of snakes overrunning its surroundings (Livy 4.59.4; Pliny *NH* 3.59, 8.104).[2] We also know of the marshes of Minturnae, at the mouth of the river Liri: here Marius, and later on Varus, searched in vain for a shelter; the sanctuary of Marica was nearby (Plut. *Mar.* 37–8; App. *B. Civ.* 4.28). The town of Atina appears to have been so called due to the diseases brought about by the poisonous effluvia of the bogs (*a morbis, qui graece atai dicuntur, quos paludis vicinitas creat*: Servius *ad Aen.* 7.630).

Campania was a very marshy region, especially along its coast: Liternum, for example, was a village situated near the swampish mouth of the river Liternus and famous for being Scipio Africanus Major's place of exile (Livy 22.6.14, 38.53.8; Val. Max. 5.3.2b; Sil. 6.653f., 7.276–9, 8.530f.; Stat. *Silv.* 4.3.65f.; Pliny *NH* 16.234; Seneca *Ep.* 51.11, 86.3ff.; see Borca 1994). Columella mentions a marsh next to Pompeii (10.135f.): it was possibly the boggy plain washed by the river Sarnus at the foot of Vesuvius and was close to the salines of Hercules (perhaps the salines at Herculaneum). In Lucania, Paestum was made unwholesome by the fens created by a watercourse stagnating just at the bottom of the walls (Strabo 6.1.1). Finally we can note that according to Servius, Velia was named after the marshes – *helē* in Greek – which surrounded it (Servius *ad Aen.* 6.359).[3]

Advantages of marshes

The examples noted above stress the presence of towns in or close to marshy areas. Any disadvantages were often out-weighed by the advantages conveyed by location, communications and trade. A strategically strong position was undoubtedly useful for any settlement and in fact swamps and marshes could play a part in providing this. The benefits at Ravenna and Alexandria have already been mentioned. At the Indian city of Sangala a ring of walls together with a swamp constituted the defensive apparatus of the site (Arr. *Anab.* 5.23; Curt. 9.1.14). The queen Semiramis, when founding Babylon, did not build fortifications in the large area over which marshes stretched (Diod. Sic. 2.7.5). These swamps spread to the west of the city as far as the walls, as well as southward, and formed an impassable defence (Arr. *Anab.* 7.17; Strabo 16.4.1; Pliny *NH* 6.27). Similar examples are numerous. In Macedonia, marshes of impenetrable depth surrounded Pella in summer as well as in winter (Livy 44.46.5–6); in Cisalpine Gaul Mantua rose in a favourable spot, protected by the meanders and bogs of the river Mincius (*Priapea* 3.1; Schol. Verg. Bern. *Ecl.* 9.29; Servius *Ecl.* 9.10: see Borca 1997d: 18ff.). Among the prodigies which occurred in 214 BC Livy recounts that at Mantua a swamp, the overflow of the Mincius, appeared bloody (Livy 24.10.7). In Sicily, there were fens in the proximity of Enna and Agrigentum, and marshy grounds performed a remarkable function of defence at Syracuse (Diod. Sic. 5.3.3; Strabo 6.2.9; Thuc. 6.101.3; Vib. Seq. *Geogr.* p. 68 Parroni; Steph. Byz. s.v. 'Syrakousai'); Diodorus Siculus (14.70–1) discusses the exhalations of these fens, along with the stench of unburied corpses, in describing the epidemic which decimated the Carthaginians, who had sacked the temple of Demeter and Cora. Earlier the swampish confined place, lacking air currents, is identified as a factor in the disease which killed many victims among the Athenian soldiers. The harmfulness of an environment diseased by stagnating waters is perceived as something physically present, almost palpable.[4] The vapours sent forth by the rotting marsh either drive men out or overwhelm them with a mantle of unbreathable air. Indeed the foul odour rising from marshes bears down on Graviscae, a town in Etruria, which therefore must literally hold up or sustain the load of the overhanging heavy air (Cato F 46 P = Servius *ad Aen.* 10.184; Rut. Namat. 1.281–2).

At Pharsalus, in Thessaly, marshes were formed by the overflow of the river Enipeus. These benefited Caesar, when fighting against Pompey, since they were impassable and precluded the possibility of being surrounded and so represented an element of great tactical importance in arraying the troops (Frontin. *Str.* 2.3.22). Cartagena also enjoyed an enviable position and was closed on the west side by a coastal bog. Unfortunately this protection was overrated by the inhabitants and turned out to be the Achilles' heel of their defences.[5] If the people of Cartagena relied too much upon the nature of the site, the inhabitants of Camarina, on the contrary, were not aware of the protection given by the fen, which shielded them from their enemies. A marsh formed by the standing waters of the river Hipparis stood adjacent to the northern side of the walls (cf. Pind. *Ol.* 5.11–12; Claudian. *De rapt. Pros.* 2.59). The marsh had dried and generated a *pestilentia*; the inhabitants then consulted Apollo's oracle in order to know whether they should reclaim it; Apollo replied and recommended them to let it alone. Yet the people of Camarina ignored this response, they dried the swamps up and, then free from the pestilence, paid the penalty to their enemies, who entered the town through the former marsh (Servius *ad Aen.* 3.701; cf. Verg. *Aen.* 3.700; Ov. *Fast.* 4.477; Sil. 14.198; Suid. s.v. 'Mē kinei Kamarinan'; Steph. Byz. s.v. 'Kamarina'; Traina 1986; Fedeli 1990: 41).

The marsh as a liminal space

At Camarina, as in other places benefiting from the nature of the site, the marsh appears to be a liminal area; it serves as a boundary, fixed by nature, to separate and protect. Simultaneously it is an environment alien to culture; ambiguous and chaotic; a space subject to divine – certainly not human – control. The people of Camarina disregard the oracular response and thus become culpable of *hybris* against the god; they decide to intervene and radically modify a natural milieu which has been excluded from reclamation;

they have been warned of the consequences: despite being an unhealthy place, it is best that culture does not prevail over the marsh. The recovery works eliminate the *pestilentia* but, fatally, it also opens up a passage for the enemies, who will destroy the town. Impious and foolish, the inhabitants have torn down the defence which secured their safety; they have usurped the deity's dominion on the marsh and they have rashly transformed a space which only nature had the power to change or remove. Witless, they have cut a way in for the enemy and have determined the worst punishment for themselves. A high price – the loss of identity – has to be paid for this inopportune modification by a transgressive culture. In its disappearance the marsh entangles the very men who are responsible for that disappearance.

The story of Camarina is indicative of the precarious equilibrium characteristic of the city–marsh relationship. The noxious animals, the effluvia, the winds interacting with the particular hydrological condition, and finally the disease caused by these factors, all contribute to the creation of a natural barrier between man and the bog. In the Romanocentric perspective, only beasts and the representatives of alien communities can feel at ease with and find shelter in marshes. It is a real swamp of humanity, made of brigands, like the Egyptian Boukoloi (Bertrand 1988),[6] and of barbarian peoples like the Gauls, the Germans and the Britons. These people choose to live in these areas and benefit by places usually considered treacherous and impenetrable (Borca 1996a; 1996e).

A cultural space *par excellence*, the city appears to be far removed from the filth of the fens. This is made apparent in the urgent warning – almost a maxim – with which Palladius firmly denounces that the marsh milieu has nothing to do with culture and human settlement. Its deleterious atmosphere and the baneful animals bred in it mean that the marsh should be avoided (1.7.4). Nevertheless, the swamp, as we have seen, is not completely driven out of the ancients' cultural and spatial horizon. The stagnating water floods and sinks through the folds of the cultural texture; in other words, there is no concrete will to eliminate marshlands totally – which, considering the technological limits of those times, would have been anyhow impractical. The construction of a road, the building of a villa, a warehouse, a theatre or a city, or the cultivation of a plot of ground, in short any kind of cultural intervention on the natural environment, needed to take into consideration the possible presence of marshes; troublesome and pestiferous perhaps, but more often than not, insuppressible neighbours.

Conclusion: Bees, men and marshes

The repellent putridity and the pernicious miasmata emanating from bogs keep away not only men, but also bees. When, in the fourth book of the *Georgics*, Virgil gives advice on the adoption of a suitable place for beekeeping, he warns against trusting a deep marsh, and places where foul odours rise from filth (Verg. *Georg.* 4.48f. with Borca 1995c). Varro suggests setting the apiary close to the farm – therefore, in a wholesome site far from swampy grounds – and where pure water is available (Varro *Rust.* 3.16.12,15,27: cf. Arist. *Hist. An.* 596b; *Geopon.* 15.2.1–4; Verg. *Georg.* 4.18–19, 25–8 with Della Corte 1984). Columella's description is more precise: the hive should be put in a position neither too hot nor excessively cold, since these insects are troubled by both conditions; bees must be kept away from the latrines, the dunghill and the bathroom because of foul odours; for the same reason it is necessary to avoid those plants whose smell is heavy and nauseous; the odour of a crab when it is burnt on the fire; and the odour rising from the filth of marshes (Columella 9.5: cf. Arist. *Hist. An.* 596b; Varro *Rust.* 3, 16; Palladius 1.36.3,5; *Geopon.* 15.3.4; Crane and Graham 1985; Crane 1994). The bees seek only the pure: they abhor all that is putrescent and there is nothing more rotten than filthy marsh mud (Varro *Rust.* 3.16.6; cf. Pliny *NH* 11.18).

Not only do bees detest and avoid bad odours, but neither can they suffer spicy fragrances and artificial scents: that is why they fly at perfumed people (Pliny *NH* 11.25; Aelian. *Hist. An.* 1.58). Hostile to luxury and ease and also to rot and putrefaction, the bee seems to have a peculiar cultural aspect: like man, it avoids both climatic (neither oppressive hot, nor icy cold: Varro *Rust.* 3.16.37; Verg. *Georg.* 4.37) and olfactory-alimentary excesses (neither the foul-smelling plants and the putrid mud, nor spices and perfumes: see Bettini 1986: 205ff.). It is not by chance that mosquitoes, marsh creatures *par excellence* and real pests (Beavis 1988: 233), together with wasps and hornets, are among the worst enemies of the bee, not to mention frogs, the most characteristic and noisy marsh animals (Varro *Rust.* 3.16.19; Aelian. *Hist. An.* 1.58; Palladius 9.6; Borca 1997e). Not only does the frog's typical habitat coincide with the biotope most adverse to the bee, but the batrachians themselves are enemies of these insects: immune from their sting, in fact, swamp frogs feed on bees (Arist. *Hist. an.* 9.189; Pliny *NH* 11.61f.; Aelian. *Hist. An.* 5.11).

The bee world is contiguous to the humanised and civilised one: men and bees, inhabitants of healthy sites, contrast with the beasts living in *pestilentes* places. The abode of often dangerous but always negatively perceived animals, the marsh environment is an ideal habitat for tormenting insects, noisy frogs and insidious snakes. In positioning an apiary, on the contrary, one must adopt the same principles employed in choosing a site appropriate for human settlement. The bee becomes a metaphor for civilised man, and is as far removed from wild nature as man is. Men and bees live on dry land, in a place situated midway between burnt and putrid, and at a suitable distance from excessive dampness and filthy marshes.

NOTES

* This chapter partly takes up some of the themes explored in previous articles: cf. Borca 1995c; 1996b; 1997c.

1 Varro's conceptions about the causes of diseases could have been influenced by Epicureanism: Phillips 1982; on marsh *pestilentia* see André 1980; Borca 1995a: 249ff., 258ff.

2 Strabo too (5.3.6) tells about a great marsh in front of Tarracina and adds: 'near Tarracina there is a canal which runs alongside the Appian Way, and is fed at numerous places by waters from the marshes and the rivers. People navigate the canal, preferably by night ... but they also navigate it by day. The boat is towed by a mule' (trans. H. L. Jones, II, 1923). We know that when Horace had to reach *Forum Appi* and the sanctuary of *Feronia*, he travelled by canal; for the Appian Way, in this area of the Pomptine marshes, must have been in precarious condition (Hor. *Sat.* 1.5).

3 *Dicta est a paludibus, quibus cingitur, quas Graeci helē dicunt. Fuit ergo 'Elia', sed accepit digammon et facta est 'Velia', ut 'Enetus Venetus'*; Servius *ad Aen.* 6.359.

4 Such a perception, entwined with that of the marsh *gravis aqua*, takes form in the concept of *gravitas loci*: see, e.g., Varro *Rust.* 1.17.2; Lucr. 6.221; Sall. *Hist.* frg. 3.96; Cic. *Att.* 11.21.2, 22.2; Hor. *Sat.* 2.6.19; Vitr. 1.4.6; Livy 23.24.11, 25.26.13, 37.23.2; Sen. *Dial.* 6.17.5, 11.7.8; *Q. Nat.* 5.10.4; *Ep.* 91.12; Tac. *Ann.* 2.85; Stat. *Theb.* 12.248.

5 I am referring to the tactics adopted by Scipio in the siege of the town in 209 BC, which were based on flood and ebb tides and on the variations of water level in the *stagnum*: cf. Livy 26.43.8, 26.45.7–46.2. For a description of the site and the capture of Cartagena cf. also Polyb. 10.9.8–10, 20.8; Sil. 15.191–250.

6 Since the second millennium BC the Nile delta had been used as a natural defence against possible enemy attacks from the sea. A peculiar *genre de vie* had developed in this area, with settlements of fishermen, hunters and herdsmen who had chosen marshes and swamps as their habitat and lived on the animal resources and fertile soil of the region. These groups could be joined by bandits and rebels; people who looked for a refuge in the labyrinthic network of lakes, channels and reeds, sometimes with the help and complicity of the local inhabitants. We know from Heliodorus' *Aethiopica* (1.5–6) that the Egyptian brigands had gathered in a region named Boukolia: here they had elected the marsh as their homeland (*patris*). Being protected by water and vegetation, the Boukoloi lived secure from any attack in a space as treacherous as they were. They inverted the cultural parameters of order, thus overturning the very idea of *patris*: it was a world populated by ugly, wicked and dreadful men who spoke and fought in a barbarous way, who did not know how to use fire for their cooking, who lived on brigandage by hunting men instead of animal prey, who could even eat human flesh. The Boukoloi's otherness is total and their anti-state, described by Heliodorus at the beginning of his novel, provides an appropriate starting-point for Charicleia's long and difficult way to Ethiopia, a land of divine wisdom at the very edges of the earth: the idealised journey leads from the negative sphere of those ferocious bandits to the perfect humanity of the blameless Ethiopians.

8

ON THE MARGINS OF THE CITY OF ROME

John R. Patterson

Introduction

This chapter examines a case-study – or perhaps better, the central case-study – for issues relating to pollution and marginality in the Roman city, namely the city of Rome itself. Although it involves discussion of literary, epigraphic and legal evidence, the main focus is topographical, as it seeks to assess what the urban layout of Rome, in particular the area which lies between the Servian and Aurelian Walls, might tell us about the activities which are, for one reason or another, excluded from the city.

Like any investigation of the topography of ancient Rome, the exercise is not without its problems. The topography of the periphery of the city in antiquity was extremely complex, and reconstructing it is made more difficult by the later occupation history of the city; the Campus Martius, for example, was among the areas most densely inhabited in mediaeval times, and continues to be almost entirely built-up today; while the Esquiline in particular was affected by major building in the later nineteenth century as the city of Rome became the capital of the Italian state. The data for building up a map of the periphery of the ancient city is therefore fragmentary and problematic. Secondly, in order to identify marginal activities, we need to establish boundaries which locate and marginalise them; as I will be demonstrating, the city of Rome simultaneously had several different boundaries relating to different spheres of human activity, both formally and informally constituted. Even those boundaries which were supposedly clearly defined, however, were in practice not always easily traced even in antiquity. The third problem is that the layout of the city, and the boundaries that defined it, changed significantly over time.

The aim of this chapter is firstly to define the different boundaries of the city, secondly to examine the types of activities which were excluded from the city by these boundaries, and thirdly to consider how far the way in which these boundaries tended to move across time had an impact on activities in the marginal zone. It concludes with a discussion of one specific area on the margins of the city, the last mile or so of the Via Appia as it approached Rome's Porta Capena from the south. Throughout the discussion it will be clear that the nature of this marginal zone was affected by considerations of what was best for the health and well-being of the inhabitants of the city. Yet this area was not just reserved for activities which were physically dangerous, or politically and ideologically inappropriate for the central spaces of civic life, and the burial of the dead. Indeed often the tombs and funerary monuments of the dead need to be placed in a broader monumental context. What I aim to show is that the topography of the periphery of the city was affected by considerations of prestige and political image-making as much as by a concern to exclude undesirable activities from the centre; but also that the interrelation of these trends led to the creation of a complex and ambiguous urban landscape on the margins of the city, which tended to subvert the political messages of monumental building.

Boundaries

Several different boundaries surrounded the city of Rome (Champlin 1982: 97). We might define them as:

- physical boundaries
- ritual boundaries
- economic boundaries
- legal boundaries

In some cases these corresponded with each other – as, for example, where the law prohibited a certain activity, such as burial, within a ritually defined boundary – but there were also some significant discrepancies, particularly during the late republic and early empire, which are of particular interest, and constitute a particular focus of this study.

Firstly, the physical boundaries, and specifically Rome's two sets of city walls, the Servian and Aurelian Walls. The Romans believed that their city had defensive walls from the beginning; one version of the founding legend of the city had it that Remus was killed when he derisively jumped over the walls of the Palatine being constructed by his brother Romulus (Livy 1.7.1; see Wiseman 1995: 9–11). Recent excavations on the northern slopes of the Palatine have revealed the remains of a wall dated to the eighth century BC, replaced by new walls in the seventh and sixth centuries, which in turn went out of use in the late sixth century, and it is tempting to associate this with Tacitus' account of the archaic boundary of the Palatine (*Annals* 12.24; see Carandini 1992; Carandini et al. 1992; Terrenato 1996; Carandini 1997: 578–80). As the city expanded to encompass more and more of the hills of Rome, we must imagine that the wall-circuit too was extended; the definitive creation of Rome's fortifications was attributed by tradition to Rome's sixth king, Servius Tullius. In recent years it has become common to ascribe the creation of this wall-circuit to the fourth century BC since we know from Livy's historical narrative that major structural work on Rome's walls took place in 378 BC (Livy 6.32; see e.g. Todd 1978: 17). This project has been identified with the phase of walling using Grotta Oscura tufa, which, since it was quarried in the territory of Veii, was only available to the Romans after their defeat of the Veientes in 396 BC. However, it is now clear that the rougher, but locally available, *cappellaccio* type of tufa was also employed in the building of the Servian Wall (as it was in other buildings clearly dated to the sixth century BC, such as the podium of the Temple of Jupiter Capitolinus) and this would suggest that some parts at least of the wall circuit may indeed date to this earlier period. Parallels from other sites in Latium also make a sixth-century date for such fortifications quite plausible (Coarelli 1995a: 20–7; Andreussi 1996: 319–20; Cifani 1997). This circuit included the central political area of the city, the Palatine and Forum, but also the Quirinal, Viminal, Esquiline, Caelian and Aventine. There were some restorations to the wall, for example after the battle of Trasimene in 217 BC, when an imminent assault on the city by Hannibal was feared (Livy 22.8.7) and then in the civil wars of the 80s BC, when Rome was besieged by Cinna and Marius (Appian, *Civil Wars* 1.66), but the circuit essentially seems to have remained the same from the sixth century BC through to the late third century AD despite the fact that the city was expanding beyond it in all directions. In some places, later buildings were built up against or on top of the Servian Wall (for example the 'Auditorium' in the Horti Maecenatis on the Esquiline); Dionysius of Halicarnassus, writing in the time of Augustus, commented that the wall was 'hard to find due to the buildings constructed around it in many areas' (4.13.5). Nevertheless, it does seem to have maintained a symbolic importance into the Imperial period (Le Gall 1991): several of the gates (for example the Porta Esquilina, Porta Caelimontana and Porta Flumentana) were rebuilt during the principate of Augustus (Coarelli 1996b; 1996d; 1996e). We hear of Nero posting guards on the wall to catch the Pisonian conspirators in AD 65 (Tacitus, *Annals* 15.58); on his return from a tour of dramatic and athletic festivals in Greece, he had a portion of the wall demolished so he could enter the city like a victorious Greek athlete (Suetonius, *Nero* 25; Dio 62.20). By contrast, Septimius Severus made a point of modestly passing though the Servian Wall on foot, when entering the city for the first time as emperor (Dio 74.1).

In the late third century AD the Romans had to think again of defending their city. Not only had it expanded to such an extent that the Servian Wall only encompassed a fraction of the built-up area, but the increasingly difficult military situation on the frontiers meant that there was a real danger of an invasion of Italy and attacks on the city itself, particularly from tribes on the Danube. In AD 270 the Alamanni, who had invaded northern Italy and caused widespread devastation, were pushed back by the emperor Aurelian, who then set about constructing a new wall-circuit for Rome (Historia Augusta,

Aurelian 21.9). This was substantially more extensive than the Servian Wall, 19 km in circumference rather than 11 km (Richmond 1930; Todd 1978: 21–45; Pisani Sartorio 1996d), and incorporated densely occupied areas which had not previously been defended, like the Janiculum and the Transtiberim region. These walls were reinforced by Maxentius in the fourth century and then again by Arcadius and Honorius at the very beginning of the fifth; they became the basis for the defences of mediaeval and renaissance Rome (Coates-Stephens 1998), and were even acting as the city's fortifications in 1870, when Italian troops entered the city through a breach in the wall near Porta Pia.

Another boundary line, of major ritual (and indeed political) significance, was the *pomerium* (Catalano 1978: 479–91; Richardson 1992: 293–6; Laurence 1993; Andreussi 1999; Beard et al. 1998, i: 177–81; ii: 93–6). This was the sacred boundary laid out by the augurs which divided the city (*urbs*) from its territory (*ager*), and marked the limit of the urban auspices (Aulus Gellius 13.14.1). However, different ancient authors had different views on the exact significance of the term and also what the *pomerium* looked like on the ground. Livy saw it as an open space on either side of the city wall (1.44.3–5), while Varro and Plutarch instead believed it was a line defining the edge of the city (Varro, *On the Latin Language* 5.143; Plutarch, *Romulus* 11.3). Tacitus describes the *pomerium* surrounding Romulus' Palatine settlement, which linked in the form of a quadrilateral the Ara Maxima of Hercules, the Altar of Consus in the Circus Maximus, the Curiae Veteres, and the shrine of the Lares; by the late Republic, the *pomerium* largely followed the line of the Servian Wall, although the Aventine continued to be excluded until the time of the emperor Claudius. This was (it seems) principally because of the hill's association with Remus' unsuccessful taking of the auspices at the time of Romulus' foundation of the city on the Palatine (Aulus Gellius 13.14.5–6), but also perhaps because of the hill's long association with the plebeian cause during the years of the 'Struggle of the Orders' (Seneca, *On the shortness of life* 13.8).

The *pomerium* was extended on several occasions from the dictatorship of Sulla onwards, but the circumstances of these initiatives, the new lines it followed, and even the identity of those responsible, remain problematic, given the contradictory and confusing nature of the literary evidence (Giardina 1997: 117–19). Extending the *pomerium* – which had, according to the myth, originally been established by Romulus – in some sense represented a kingly act, an expansion and re-foundation of the city, so it was confined to those who in practice held unfettered power in the city, principally the emperors but also the dictators Sulla and Julius Caesar (Griffin 1962: 109–10). Despite statements in Tacitus and Dio to this effect, it seems likely that Augustus did not expand the *pomerium* himself, given that such an action is not mentioned in the *Res Gestae* or as a precedent in the *Lex de imperio Vespasiani* (Boatwright 1986: 19). The best-attested extensions of the *pomerium* are those of Claudius and Vespasian. Claudius' revision of the line of the *pomerium* was the most thorough-going, reflecting both that emperor's interest in the traditions and rituals of the Etruscans (Suetonius *Claudius* 42; Levick 1990: 18) and his desire to commemorate in a striking visual way his invasion of Britain, which itself was largely motivated by his previous lack of military experience (Levick 1990: 137–48; Stewart 1995). He incorporated the Aventine within the ritual bounds of the city for the first time (Aulus Gellius 13.14.5–6), together with the southern part of the Campus Martius and large areas to the north and east of the city. The new *pomerium* was marked out by a series of *cippi* (pillars) nearly 2 m in height (at least 139 of them), inscribed with the legend *auctis populi Romani finibus* ('the frontiers of the Roman people having been extended'). A triumphal arch erected across the Via Flaminia to commemorate Claudius' victories in Britain (De Maria 1988: 280–2; Barrett 1991; Rodriguez Almeida 1993a) seems also to have marked the point at which the new *pomerium* crossed the road (Rodriguez Almeida 1981: 124–6). Several ancient discussions of the *pomerium* (including that of Gellius) relate the right to extend it to achievements in extending the frontiers of Rome, although there was evidently some controversy at the time of Claudius' extension as to whether overseas dominions counted for this purpose, or whether the new land acquired had to be in Italy (Boatwright 1984–5; Giardina 1997: 122–8 discussing Seneca, *On the shortness of life* 13.8). Expanding the *pomerium* was one of the privileges specifically granted to Vespasian under the *Lex de imperio Vespasiani* (*CIL* 6.930 = *ILS* 244, 14–16), and the expansion was implemented in AD 75; Hadrian's intervention, by contrast, was limited to re-establishing the pre-existing line of the *pomerium* and restoring the *cippi* which marked its route through the city (Labrousse 1937: 172–3). According to the *Historia Augusta*, Aurelian expanded it to tie in with his new wall-circuit, but only after having defeated Zenobia of Palmyra and the Goths so he could plausibly claim to have expanded the frontiers of the empire (*Aurelian* 21.10–11, with Syme 1983).

This ritual boundary of the city was itself paralleled further out by a series of shrines some five or six miles along the roads leading out from Rome, such as those of Terminus on the Via Laurentina, Fortuna Muliebris on the Via Latina and Dea Dia on the Via Campana, which formed the boundary of the territory of the archaic city. It continued to be marked by a series of processions and festivals, involving members of Rome's senatorial order, even into the imperial period when Rome's territory extended across the known world (Scheid 1987; Laurence 1993: 83–4).

A separate economic frontier to the city of Rome can be identified in the form of a customs-boundary, with 37 gates, which allowed taxes to be levied on goods to be sold within the city. Stone pillars have been discovered on the Via Flaminia, Via Salaria and Via Asinaria, recording how the boundary was consolidated by Marcus Aurelius and Commodus in the late 170s AD, but it is first attested in AD 74 (Pliny, *Natural History* 3.65–6; see Palmer 1980; Frézouls 1987: 384–5) and may even date back to the time of Augustus, who divided the city into fourteen regions (Suetonius, *Augustus* 30: see Nicolet 1991, 189–207). In many places the customs-boundary also formed the basis of the line adopted by Aurelian for his new wall-circuit and *pomerium* (the pillars were located near to the sites of several of the Aurelianic gates), although the territory encompassed by the new wall-circuit was overall significantly smaller than that enclosed within the fourteen regions (Frézouls 1987: 373–4).

A less precise form of boundary, but nevertheless an extremely important one, was the concept of the *continentia aedificia* ('built-up area') devised by the Roman jurists. This covered those areas which were not included within the Servian Wall or the *pomerium*, but were densely occupied, and so needed in some way to be defined as part of the city, in particular where legal responsibility for administration had to be established, or where protection against nuisances and anti-social activities was required. As Dionysius of Halicarnassus noted, it was difficult to tell where the city ended and the countryside began (4.13.4). In the late Republic such legislation was framed so as to equate the built-up area with a distance of a mile from the city walls, as for example when choosing a panel of men domiciled at Rome (*Lex repetundarum* 13, with Crawford 1996: 99) or in defining the responsibilities of the aediles (*Tabula Heracleensis* 20, with Crawford 1996: 380). By the third century AD, however, the mile was defined as beginning at the limit of the built-up area (*Digest* 50.16.154) and the definition of the city had thus become sufficiently flexible to reflect the changing situation on the ground as the city grew (Frézouls 1987: 381–2). In a similar way, the jurisdiction of the *praetor urbanus* extended to a line a hundred miles from the city, beyond which was the responsibility of the praetorian prefect (Robinson 1992: 183).

Exclusions

In this way we can see that the city of Rome was surrounded by a number of different boundaries, each pertaining to a specific aspect of human activity – ritual, military and economic. These boundaries were often significant in legal terms, too, since they frequently defined areas in which specific activities were allowed or forbidden; and this is reflected in the different types of activities that we can detect taking place beyond the city walls and beyond the customs boundary. These include political and military gatherings, cult-sites associated with alien religions and hazardous and offensive activities of various kinds; but most importantly the dangers to the physical health of the citizens and the ritual well-being of the city posed by the dead.

The regulations relating to the *pomerium* provide the clearest illustration of this pattern (Laurence 1993: 80–1). Its role as the ritual boundary between the *urbs* and the *ager* was symbolised by the fact that a magistrate who had taken the auspices within the city was obliged to take them again once he had stepped across the *pomerium*. Cicero describes how the consuls of 162 BC had to resign when it was discovered that Ti. Sempronius Gracchus, who had been presiding over the assembly at which they had been elected, had failed to carry out this procedure and therefore the consuls had not been properly elected (Cicero, *On the nature of the gods* 2.10–1). The *pomerium* also represented the distinguishing line between the city, peaceful and subject to civilian administration, and the territory beyond, potentially hostile and the concern of military commanders. The powers of magistrates, therefore, were in several cases defined by reference to the *pomerium*. The authority of the tribunes of the plebs, for example, seems normally to have been restricted to within the *pomerium* (Dionysius of Halicarnassus 8.87.7; Dio 51.19.6); conversely, the *imperium proconsulare* allocated to a military commander or provincial governor lapsed when he crossed the *pomerium* and entered the city. When the Senate needed to meet with a commander in the field who was to retain his *imperium*, the meeting had to take place in a location beyond the *pomerium*, typically in the temple of Bellona or that of Apollo near the Circus Flaminius; here too the senators met with ambassadors of hostile states in a place for informal gatherings known as a *senaculum* (Festus 470L; Bonnefond-Coudry 1989: 137–60; Coarelli 1999b).

Some areas within the periphery of the city therefore had strong military associations. The Roman army, like its commanders, was during the Republic not allowed inside the *pomerium* under normal circumstances, except when a triumphal procession had been formally authorised by the Senate; so it was on the Campus Martius, outside the *pomerium*, that the army would assemble before a triumph or prior to setting off on campaign (Varro, *On agriculture* 3.2.4). It was also on the Campus Martius that the meetings of the *comitia centuriata* would take place, since its organisation reflected the Roman people assembled for war (Aulus Gellius 15.27.5; Lintott 1999: 55–6). Under the Empire soldiers were deployed in the capital on a much more regular basis than they had been under the Republic, to protect the person of the emperor (Durry 1968: 274; Campbell 1984: 109–20) and to maintain public order. The camp of the Praetorian Guard and of the city's police force, the urban cohorts, was established on the Viminal by Tiberius in AD 23. Located outside the Servian Wall and the *pomerium* (Lissi Caronna 1993b), and so not formally within the city, this could simultaneously be represented as keeping the soldiers away from 'the enticements of the city' (Tacitus, *Annals* 4.2) and respecting the concerns of traditionalist senators, but was close enough to the centre of Rome for rapid mobilisation should the situation demand it (Robinson 1992: 181–8; Nippel 1995: 91–5). Other military barracks, like those of the Equites Singulares on the Lateran (Buzzetti 1993) and of soldiers in transit to the provincial armies on the Caelian (Lissi Caronna 1993a) were similarly located outside the Servian Walls; but, like the camp of the Praetorians, they were included within Aurelian's wall-circuit as the defence of the city from outside threats became paramount.

It has sometimes been argued that foreign cults were subject to a blanket exclusion from the area within the *pomerium*, but it appears that lack of space for the establishing of new cult-centres was a more serious problem (Ziolkowski 1992: 278). On the other hand, it is clear that some categories of worship were on different occasions banned from the ritual precincts of the city – for example the *di inferi*, deities of the underworld (Festus 478L) – and specific measures were taken to exclude Egyptian cults from the *pomerium* by Augustus following earlier legislation (Dio 53.2.4, cf. 40.47.4) and then by Agrippa, who extended the ban to a distance of one mile of the city (Dio 54.6.6).

Perhaps the most significant exclusion from the city, however, is that of the dead. The Twelve Tables state clearly that 'a dead man shall not be burned or buried within the city' (Cicero, *On the laws* 2.58), and there were very few exceptions. A handful of families, such as those of P. Valerius Publicola (Fontana 1999) and C. Fabricius Luscinus (Oriolo 1999) had the right to be buried inside the city, though in the imperial period this seems to have been little exercised; and Trajan was buried at the foot of his column (Eutropius, *Breviarium* 8.5.2; see Labrousse 1937: 191–2). Thus virtually all burials took place outside the *pomerium*. This rule was of major importance in determining the appearance of Rome's periphery, for it was here that rich and poor alike were buried (see Hope, in this volume). The wealthy tended to be buried in individual or family tombs, which were typically located near to roads, and became features of the suburban landscape in their own right; this was especially apparent in the second and first centuries BC, when increasing aristocratic competition led to the building of more and more impressive tombs, like that of Caecilia Metella, which was situated on a high point on the Appian Way (Toynbee 1971: 118–30; von Hesberg 1994: 32–50). The poorest inhabitants of Rome were buried in public pits on the Esquiline and Viminal (Bodel 1994: 38–52; Kyle 1998: 163–69); under the Empire the burial of the modestly affluent was often in *columbaria* built by wealthy individuals for their slaves and freedmen, or by *collegia* which provided burial as one of the privileges of membership (Toynbee 1971: 113–16; Patterson 1992). The *libitinarii*, Rome's undertakers, were based at the grove of Libitina outside the Porta Esquilina (Bodel 1994: 13–18; and in this volume); an important document from Puteoli, which most likely also reflects Roman practice, demonstrates that they were allowed in the city only when collecting corpses or inflicting punishments, and had to wear a dark-coloured cap so they could be easily identified and avoided (*AE* 1971 88; Bodel 1994: 72–80). The Roman authorities were concerned to reduce the health risks associated with the presence of unburied corpses in the city (Bodel 1994: 36–7; and in this volume), but it was also considered important to control the practice of cremation, which was the most widely used means of disposing of the dead in the late republic and early empire (Morris 1992: 31–69). Cicero suggests that this was because of the risks posed by fires, rather than religious scruples as we might otherwise imagine (*On duties* 2.58). The *Lex Coloniae Genetivae* from Urso in Spain banned cremations from within half a mile of that city (ch. 74, in Crawford 1996) and a measure passed in 38 BC prohibited the practice within two miles of the city of Rome (Dio 48.43.3), which similarly imply that practical hazards were the main concern of the authorities.

Other activities considered hazardous or detrimental to the well-being of the citizens were also confined to the periphery of the city. The *Lex Coloniae Genetivae* banned large tile-factories from urban centres, again presumably because of the danger of fire caused by the kilns (ch. 76, with Crawford 1996: 438); under the empire many of these were located on the west side of the Tiber, on the Vatican and in the vicinity of the Via Aurelia, Via Cornelia and Via Triumphalis (Petracca and Vigna 1985; Morel 1987: 131). It also appears that some activities involving noxious smells were located on the margins of the city (Morel 1987: 129–33) – the club-house of the *coriarii* or tanners was located in Transtiberim, on the other side of the Tiber from the centre of Rome (Loane 1938: 77–9; Pronti 1993; Bollmann 1997: 225; 1998: 272–3), together with their workshops (Martial 6.93; Juvenal 14.203; Scobie 1986: 419) – although similarly malodorous fulleries seem to have been more widely distributed across the city. Wild animals for exhibition at the games were kept in the *vivarium*, an enclosure which was incorporated in the wall of Aurelian near the Porta Praenestina and incorporated in Aurelian's wall (Procopius, *Gothic War* 1.22.10, 1.23.13–23), though of course the games themselves took place in the very centre of the city, in the Circus or Colosseum.

In the same way, it is clear that the aediles, responsible for keeping the streets of the city clean, made arrangements for the removal of all kinds of rubbish from the urban centre to the periphery (Robinson 1992: 69–73); special privileges were in force to allow wagons carrying *stercus* (whether this means specifically 'excrement' or 'refuse' in a more general sense is debated) to circulate within the city during the hours of daylight (*Tabula Heracleensis* 66–7, in Crawford 1996; see Robinson 1992: 122–3; Bodel 1994: 30). Tacitus tells us that Messalina tried to escape from her husband Claudius by hiding in a wagon carying *purgamenta hortorum* (garden refuse?) along the Via Ostiensis (*Annals* 11.32; see Beard 1998: 28), and presumably much of this rubbish ended up on the outskirts of the city. Nero decided to dump the debris from the great fire of AD 64 in the marshes near Ostia (Tacitus, *Annals* 15.43). The human waste was potentially useful as manure (Columella 10.84–5, 11.3.12: see Scobie 1986: 413–14) for the market-gardens which surrounded the city (Carandini 1988; Morley 1996: 83–90), but legal texts and inscriptions alike suggest that illicit dumping was also a problem (*Digest* 43.10.1.5; Bodel 1994: 32–5).

As well as the marginalisation of activities or substances ritually considered impure, and those activities which were undesirable for reasons of health, hygiene and well-being, economic considerations also influenced the organisation of the periphery of the city. The creation of a customs-boundary must have had some specific effects – for example, inducing traders to set up depots for the import or distribution of produce beyond the boundary rather than within it, to reduce their liability to customs duties. This is particularly true of the reaches of the Tiber just above and below the city. The Cellae Vinariae Nova et Arruntiana, wine warehouses on the right bank of the Tiber, must have been located just at the edge of the city (Rodriguez Almeida 1993e); the Aurelian wall was built through them, bringing activity there to an end after AD 271 (Palmer 1980: 224; Cozza 1986: 111–12). Other port facilities located above the city similarly dealt in wine being brought down the Tiber from Umbria and inland Etruria. The wine-depot at Septem Caesares, below the city, served the same purpose for produce being brought upstream (Palmer 1980: 224; 1981: 368–9; Lega 1999). Several livestock markets in the city are known by name; unfortunately in most cases their position in the city is unclear, although it does appear that in late antiquity the Forum Suarium was located close to the Via Flaminia in the vicinity of Aurelian's Temple of the Sun, which was itself used for the storage of wine collected by the state in the form of customs dues, prior to its distribution to the people of Rome (Historia Augusta, *Aurelian* 48.4; see Palmer 1980: 220; Torelli 1992: 121). Both of these complexes were easily accessible from Aurelian's Porta Flaminia, Rome's gateway to the north, and from the Tiber ports.

Similarly, Coarelli has shown that luxury food markets, the *macella*, were moved towards the south-east corner of the city in the imperial period (Coarelli 1986: 41–3). The central *macellum*, which had itself been created behind the Forum Romanum in the third century BC (De Ruyt 1983: 158–63; Coarelli 1985: 149–55; Pisani Sartorio 1996a), was restructured in the Flavian period (Tortorici 1991: 44), and disappeared under Nerva. The Macellum Liviae, completed in 7 BC, was located just outside the Porta Esquilina (De Ruyt 1983: 163–72; Pisani Sartorio 1996b), and Nero's Macellum Magnum was built on the Caelian hill (De Ruyt 1983: 172–84; Carignani et al. 1990; Pisani Sartorio 1996c). Presumably as well as reflecting the dense occupation of these areas of the city, this must in part be related to the fact that many of the farms producing vegetables and small animals for the Roman market were located beyond the south-east quadrant of the city, well supplied with water from aqueducts and manure from the city, and with easy access to the markets by road (Carandini 1988: 339–57; Morley 1996: 83–107). However, considerations of appropriateness may also have played a part in the location of the *macella*, as they may have done in consigning other activities to the margins of the city. Varro, apparently discussing the replacement of butchers' shops by silversmiths' in the Forum of the late fourth century BC, comments that 'the dignity of the Forum' was thereby enhanced (quoted in Nonius Marcellus 853L, with Coarelli 1985: 141–3), but he may of course be reflecting the perceptions of his own time more than those of the fourth century. The building of the imperial fora, from Julius Caesar onwards, certainly contributed to the divorce of ceremonial and commercial activity within public space in Rome (Morel 1987: 137–9; Purcell 1995, 333–5). Not only were there some activities which members of the Roman elite considered inappropriate for the central spaces of civic life, but evidence from Pompeii suggests that this ideology did indeed have practical consequences in terms of the distribution of activities in the city, with brothels and taverns concentrated in areas away from public buildings and the Forum (Seneca, *On the good life* 7.3, with Wallace-Hadrill 1995).

Considerations of appropriateness or nuisance are of course much less clearly definable than the clearly demarcated line represented by the *pomerium* or city wall, and their effects less easy for us to identify. Perceptions of what was appropriate or tolerable may have varied according to the social class of the viewer, among other factors; and the degree to which exclusion was implemented evidently varied in practice. Cicero, for example, clearly thought that the smells and appearance of drains were offensive: he refers to the concern of architects to keep away from the eyes and noses of a householder 'those fluid substances with which necessarily an element of offensiveness is associated' (Cicero, *On the nature of the gods* 2.141). Nevertheless, in many urban dwellings drainage was rudimentary, and a fullery, for example, might be located close to a wealthy *domus*. Some nuisances were also taken more seriously than others by the Roman authorities: the risks from fire impinged on the safety of public as well as private buildings, as repeated disastrous fires at Rome had shown, and this helps to explain the legally enforced restrictions on cremation and tile-works in the city.

Flexible boundaries and shifting exclusions

The continuing expansion of the city, the advent of the principate, which brought with it the transformation of the political system, and the various initiatives undertaken by individual emperors, meant that even the supposedly fixed linear boundaries of Rome did not always stay where they were first established. Sometimes they might be moved to reflect the changing situation within the city, though this could be done more easily in some cases than others. Boundaries defined by reference to the *continentia aedificia* were much more flexible than the *pomerium*, the movement of which had major political and religious implications. Nevertheless, regulations relating to magistracies and the limits of their authority were changed on several occasions to reflect the new requirements of the principate (Laurence 1993: 81). In 30 BC Augustus was granted the right to hold his tribunician power both inside the city and up to a mile outside it (Dio 51.17.6; see Boatwright

1986: 24); in 23 BC he was made proconsul for life, without the obligation to lay down his office whenever he entered the city (Dio 53.32.5). As we have seen, the *pomerium* itself was moved on several occasions during the late republican and imperial periods, which meant that sites and activities which might originally have been located outside the city – cemeteries in particular – were subsequently found to be within it. This problem was particularly acute in the case of the mass graves just outside the Porta Esquilina, which seem to have been covered over with a thick deposit of earth and debris early in the first century BC, presumably because the burial ground was becoming a squalid health hazard as habitation extended beyond the Servian wall (Bodel 1994: 45–7). Similar operations were conducted later in the century when Maecenas established his *horti* further to the south, and transformed the graveyard into an attractive park (Horace, *Satires* 1.8, 8–16; see Bodel 1994: 50–4). As palaces and ceremonial public spaces came to take over much of the centre of the city, the housing of the rich tended to move to the periphery of Rome. This process can already be detected with the creation of the *horti* of the late Republic (Wallace-Hadrill 1998), but it was accelerated by the fire of AD 64 and the building of Nero's Domus Aurea (Eck 1997); areas like the Esquiline were 'gentrified' and the poor, their tombs, and the detritus of the city moved elsewhere, complicating still further the topography of the periphery.

Perhaps most dramatic in its impact on the organisation of the city was the creation of Aurelian's wall-circuit and new *pomerium*, which at a stroke meant that large numbers of monumental tombs were brought within the city. In fact we owe the survival of many of these monuments to the creation of the new walls, since their hurried construction meant that many tombs were incorporated within gateways or towers, most notably the tomb of Eurysaces the baker at the Porta Maggiore and the Pyramid of Cestius at the Porta Ostiensis. The subterranean tomb of the Aurelii on the Esquiline, though some distance from the wall itself, was abandoned in the late third century AD once enclosed within the new boundary (Bisconti 1999). In some cases the reorganisation of space is even more striking; the tomb of Julius Achilles, who was of equestrian rank and acted as superintendent of the Ludus Magnus, the gladiatorial training school near the Colosseum, was set up in the late third century AD just south of the Baths of Caracalla, shortly before the Aurelian wall was built; his sarcophagus is dated by stylistic criteria to the period AD 265–70 (Avetta 1985: 57–8). By the mid-fourth century AD, however, we find a luxurious house, complete with a bath-complex and mosaic of charioteers, being built directly on top of Julius' tomb (Avetta 1985: 42). The ancient tomb of the Scipios (for which see below) suffered the same fate at some point in the third or fourth century, though whether before or after the building of the new wall-circuit is unclear (Zevi 1999: 281). Presumably this reflects not only the disappearance of tombs with the advent of the new *pomerium*, but also the spread of aristocratic housing from the centre to the periphery of the city. After 270, however, there may also have been an increased demand for housing *within* the new city wall, for the sake of security. The case of Julius Achilles' tomb illustrates perfectly the complexity of the situation between the two walls, and the extent to which change could take place over time; as the city's boundaries were moved, the nature of the periphery changed too. One additional minor change resulting from the establishment of Aurelian's wall-circuit, which nevertheless indicates its impact on concepts of space within the city, is that the portion of the Via Flaminia now within the city took a new name, the Via Lata. It was now an urban rather than a consular road (Patterson forthcoming b).

Approaching the city: the Via Appia

In examining the periphery of the city, we need to think not only in terms of those people departing from the city, and the activities which were for different reasons excluded from the centre, but also the impact of the marginal areas on those *arriving* at the city, and the ways in which leading republican senators and emperors alike used the *suburbium* of the city as a monumental entrance to the imperial capital. An examination of the initial stages of the Via Appia illustrates the multiplicity of activities taking place along this major entrance-way to the city. As we will see, there was a particularly close relationship between the roads and the construction of tombs, but the relationship between road-building and the construction of public monuments is also worthy of note.

The Via Appia, constructed to link Rome with Campania in 312 BC, was the first Roman road to take the name of its builder, the censor Appius Claudius Caecus, and had very strong historical associations: Statius called it the 'queen of roads' (*Silvae* 2.1.12: see Wiseman 1970, contra Radke 1973; Patterson forthcoming a for further bibliography). The road not only plays an important part in narratives of Appius' censorship (Livy 9.29.5–7; Diodorus 20.36.2) and official commemorations (for example his *elogium* in the Forum of Augustus: *Inscriptiones Italiae* XIII 3.79 = *CIL* I^2 p. 192, ix–x = *ILS* 54) but it is even referred to in Cicero's attack on Clodia in his *Pro Caelio*, where the orator calls up the figure of Appius to remonstrate with his descendant. 'Was it for this I built a road, that you should make use of it in the company of other women's husbands … ?' (*Pro Caelio* 34). The Appia ran originally to Capua, but it was then extended to Beneventum (probably after the creation of the Latin colony there in 268 BC), Tarentum and finally to Brundisium, where a colony was founded in 244 BC, and which became a major port for communications with the East (Coarelli 1988: 37–8; Uggeri 1990: 21–4).

The starting-point of the road was the Porta Capena in the Servian Wall, and the Appia led south-east past the temple of Mars, a mile away, which had been founded in 388 BC (Livy 6.5.7; see Richardson 1992: 244–5). It is very likely that it followed a pre-existing local road connecting Rome and the Alban Hills (Livy 7.39.16); but the fact that a series of important tombs was constructed in its vicinity from the early third century onwards indicates the importance of the development of the route for this part of the *suburbium* (Purcell 1987). The tomb of P. Cornelius Scapula was located some 400 metres from the road, and most probably predates Appius' work (Pisani Sartorio and Quilici Gigli 1987–8), but the monument of L. Cornelius Scipio Barbatus (consul 298 BC), constructed on a by-road connecting the Appia and the nearby Via Latina early in the third century, must owe its position to the new road, which was additionally 'paved with squared stones' between the Temple of Mars and the Porta Capena in 296 BC (Livy 10.23.11–12).

The son of Scipio Barbatus, L. Cornelius Scipio (consul in 259 BC) was buried in the same tomb as his father. His sarcophagus commemorates his achievements, including his capture of the city of Aleria in Corsica, and his dedication of a temple to the Tempestates (storms) (*CIL* I^2 9 = *ILS* 3). This was vowed when Scipio's fleet was surprised by a storm off the Corsican coast, during the First Punic War (Ovid, *Fasti* 6.193–4; see Ziolkowski 1992: 162–4). The precise location of the temple of the Tempestates is unfortunately not known, but since it was located in the first Augustan region of the city, not far from the temple of Mars, it must have been in the vicinity of the Appia, and is most likely to have been situated near the Scipios' family tomb. If this supposition is correct, it is very striking that we find the Scipios building both a tomb and a temple in the same area on the outskirts of the city, and this relationship is paralleled by the case of the temple of Honos and Virtus, which was located just outside the Porta Capena. The temple of Honos was probably dedicated by Q. Fabius Maximus Rullianus in the late fourth century BC (Palombi 1996). M. Claudius Marcellus, the conqueror of Syracuse, vowed a temple to Virtus next door to it (Livy 27.25.6–10) and the temple was eventually dedicated by his son in 205 BC (Livy 29.11.13). Both father and son were buried in the family mausoleum nearby, together with a third member of the family, consul in 152 BC, who erected statues of all three men on the monument with the inscription 'three Marcelli, nine times consul' (Asconius 12C). Here too, tomb-building and temple-building on the part of a major aristocratic family are taking place in a location just outside the Servian Wall. Other aristocrats buried in the area included Atilius Calatinus, another general of the First Punic War, and members of the Metellus and Servilius families were all buried close to the Appia (Cicero, *Tusculans* 1.13).

This clustering around the Appia meant that the tombs of these aristocratic families, although in theory removed from the city, in fact combined with the temples and other monuments constructed by these families to create a competitive arena as significant in its own way as areas like the Forum or the Campus Martius at the very centre of the city. The original tomb monuments seem to have been comparatively restrained in scale and appearance (von Hesberg 1994: 33), but in the mid-second century the tomb of the Scipios was rebuilt with a monumental façade more impressive to passers-by (Coarelli 1972: 62–82), at around the same time as the tomb of the Claudii Marcelli was being embellished. Just as the houses, temples and basilicas within the city reflected the rivalries of the aristocracy, so did the tombs and temples outside it (Patterson 2000: 31–45). Military success was of central importance to the monuments of the area: the *elogia* of the Scipios commemorated their conquests, the temples of the Tempestates and Virtus are both related to major Roman victories, and the temple of Mars was the focus of ceremonies connected with the departure of military expeditions (Livy 7.23.3). Some of the treasures looted from Syracuse when that city was sacked by Rome in 212 BC, including a globe designed by Archimedes, were displayed in the temple of Honos and Virtus (Livy 25.40.1–3; Cicero, *On the Republic* 1.21). The effect must have been to impress upon the visitor coming from the south, who entered the city through the Porta Capena, the extent of Roman military conquests. A speech by T. Manlius Torquatus in Livy specifically makes this point – that if Hiero of Syracuse, a one-time ally, were to rise from the dead, the first thing he would see on entering Rome 'in the vestibule of the city, almost at the gate' would be the spoils of his native city (Livy 26.32.4); the Porta Capena was a particularly appropriate location in this case, given that this is precisely where the overland traveller from Sicily would arrive in Rome. A *senaculum* like that at the temple of Bellona was set up at the Porta Capena (Festus 470L) and it was here that the Senate met, outside the *pomerium*, to agree a strategy after the disastrous defeat at the battle of Cannae, presumably so that they could confer with commanders with *imperium* operating in southern Italy (Livy 23.32.2–3; Coarelli 1999b).

The stretch of the Via Appia just outside the Porta Capena continued to be of major importance under the emperors. The gate itself was clearly of great significance in Augustus' perception of the city – *regio I* within Augustus' reorganisation of the city was that around the Porta Capena, and in late antiquity it seems to have taken on the name of the gate (Nicolet 1991: 196–7; Coarelli 1996c). Although the main focus of Augustus' own road-building activity was on the Via Flaminia 'since he was going to lead an army out by that route' (Dio 53.22.1; *Res Gestae* 20.5; Suetonius, *Augustus* 30.1), and it was close to the Flaminia that his own Mausoleum was located, together with the Horologium and Ara Pacis, milestones attest some limited work on the Appia too during his reign (Uggeri 1990: 26). Dio tells us that arches were built to honour Augustus at Brundisium and in the Forum at Rome following the battle of Actium (Dio 51.19.1). In 19 BC, the Senate set up an altar of Fortuna Redux near the Porta Capena to commemorate Augustus' safe return to the city from Syria after an expedition which culminated in the diplomatic 'victory' over the Parthians and the restoration to

Rome of the standards taken from Crassus' defeated army in 53 BC; an annual sacrifice was to take place there (*Res Gestae* 11: Coarelli 1995b). This can be seen as a precursor of the Ara Pacis set up on the Via Flaminia to commemorate Augustus' safe return from Spain and Gaul (Torelli 1982: 28–9); Augustus' achievement as conqueror of the East is thus reflected in the monuments set up on the Appia, and his northern victories on the Flaminia. Ceremonies connected with the return of an emperor to the city continued to take place in the area just outside the Porta Capena, as we have seen; the Mutatorium Caesaris, apparently the place where emperors changed from military to civilian dress on returning to the city, is known from the Severan Marble Plan to have been located not far from the gate, opposite the site of the Baths of Caracalla (Pisani Sartorio 1996e). The arch commemorating the German victories of Drusus, father of the emperor Claudius, after his death in 9 BC (Suetonius, *Claudius* 1.3), seems to have been close to the temple of Mars, again emphasising the strong military associations of this part of the urban landscape (De Maria 1988: 273; Pisani Sartorio 1993).

Similarly, we know of arches honouring Trajan and Lucius Verus located in *regio I*, which are most likely to have been situated on the Via Appia itself (De Maria 1988: 298–302; Palombi 1993a; 1993b); both emperors were distinguished for their victories against the Parthians, receiving the title 'Parthicus', as well as for their work on the Appia itself and related road-network. As part of a major programme of road-building works Trajan had initiated major improvements on the Appia itself (Galen 10.633K), with a new cutting at Tarracina and the institution of a major new road, the Via Traiana between Beneventum and Brundisium, which took his own name, and was commemorated with another arch which still survives at Benevento. Similarly, Verus may have been responsible for extending the Via Traiana from Brundisium to Hydruntum, which he used as his point of departure for his Parthian campaigns (Uggeri 1990: 27).

The most striking examples of imperial activity at the beginning of the Appia, though, are those of Septimius Severus and his successor Caracalla. Severus sought to legitimise his new authority, won in the civil war of the AD 190s, by reference to Augustus, the archetypical victor of civil war and restorer of order in the state. The arch of Severus in the Forum Romanum, for example, bears an inscription honouring him 'on account of the restoration of the state' (*CIL* 6.1033 = *ILS* 425), and he celebrated the Ludi Saeculares in AD 203 as Augustus had in 17 BC (Birley 1988: 155–9). As part of Severus' rebuilding of the Palatine, he constructed a massive nymphaeum known as the Septizodium (or Septizonium). Unfortunately, most of the monument was demolished in 1589, but Renaissance drawings and recent archaeological excavations have allowed us to reconstruct what it may have been like with some certainty. The *Historia Augusta* tells us that 'when he built the Septizodium, Severus had no other idea than that his building should meet those arriving from Africa' (*Septimius Severus* 24.3), believing (rightly or wrongly) that Severus designed the structure with the intention of reminding the viewer of his own African origin: he had been born at Lepcis Magna, and apparently retained 'an African accent' (*Septimius Severus* 19.9–10, with Birley 1988: 35). In any case, Severus had been successful in campaigns against the Parthians, which were depicted on his arch in the Forum (Historia Augusta, *Septimius Severus* 15–16), and he also improved the Via Appia (Uggeri 1990: 25). Just as the Porta Capena was the starting-point for Augustus' new scheme of regions, so the Porta Capena and the Via Appia determined the orientation of the Severan Marble Plan of Rome, occupying a position in the middle at the top of the map (Carettoni et al. 1960: 231). Severus' successor, Caracalla, built the great bath-complex which lay adjacent to the Appia just south of the Porta Capena, together with a new access road, the Via Nova, which was laid out parallel to the Appia (Historia Augusta, *Caracalla* 9.9). Again the approach to the south of the city was embellished, as the aqueduct supplying the baths crossed the Appia and provided a grand entrance-way to the city in the form of a new arch, which perhaps also commemorated Caracalla's own campaigns against the Parthians (De Maria 1988: 309–10).

The last mile or so of the Via Appia was clearly perceived as being a location of prestige and importance in the city. Under the Republic, monumental tombs commemorated distinguished aristocratic families, and temples recalled their victories over Rome's enemies; the emperors too were keen to provide a monumental entrance-way to the city for a road which was of crucial strategic importance in linking Rome with Brundisium, the main port for the East. At the same time they commemorated their own victories with a series of monumental arches which recalled the conquest of peoples to the south and to the east; victory over Egypt or the Parthians was most appropriately commemorated in this sector of the city. It is doubtless no accident that when in 1937 Mussolini erected an ancient obelisk taken from the Ethiopian city of Axum to commemorate his victories in Abyssinia, the Piazza di Porta Capena was the location chosen (D'Onofrio 1967: 309–12). Extending the *pomerium* was one way of commemorating the expansion of the empire – as the case of Claudius in particular shows – but the construction of honorific arches and other monuments on the approaches of the city had a similar effect; and would have had a specific audience in the form of the hordes of ambassadors and delegates who continually visited Rome on public business.

Conclusion

It has been estimated that perhaps 10 per cent of Aurelian's wall-circuit consists of reused buildings, so the wall itself provides a snapshot of the periphery of Rome in AD 271. As well as tombs, it incorporated houses, cisterns, aqueducts, military barracks, the Vivarium, and imperial residences such as the Sessorium and adjacent Amphitheatrum Castrense (Richmond 1930: 1–15; Pisani Sartorio 1996d: 294–5). Similarly, the Transtiberim district, which lay outside the *pomerium* until the time of Aurelian, was by the third century AD occupied by a dense network of houses, apartment blocks, workshops, port facilities, gardens, tombs, temples and other buildings (Palmer 1981; Coarelli 1992). The mixture is illustrated by an inscription which records a dispute over the boundaries of an *insula* and a tomb (*CIL* 6.10250 = *ILS* 8363, with Palmer 1981: 381). Excavations carried out in the vicinity of Porta Pia likewise revealed a landscape of villas, industrial establishments, quarries, tombs and tomb-gardens (Bird et al. 1993; Gilkes et al. 1994).

The periphery of the city was especially characterised by activities that were for various legal, social and political reasons banished from the urban centre. Religious considerations and concerns about hygiene forbade the burial of the dead within the city, and political responsibilities were circumscribed by its boundaries; the *comitia centuriata* had to meet outside the *pomerium*, and here also many military installations were located in the imperial period. The institution of a customs boundary led to a concentration of commercial activities on the edge of the city. Noxious or hazardous activities, damaging to the health of the citizens or endangering their safety, might be excluded from the built-up area, and the way in which these were defined reflected the priorities of the Roman authorities. The category of activities which, while not illegal, were nevertheless considered for one reason or another inappropriate for the very centre of the city, gradually increased from the mid-republic through to the imperial period, when much of Rome's core was given over to the Palace and to the ceremonial space of the imperial Fora.

At the same time, those activities which had for economic reasons to take place as close as was feasible to the city tended to converge on the periphery together with those activities which were excluded. For example, perishable vegetables, and animals and birds for the table, needed to be grown or raised close to Rome in order to minimise delays in transporting them to market, and the small-scale estates which specialised in these products relied on a labour force derived from the city (Carandini 1988: 340–1). These conflicting demands both raised the price of land on the outskirts – already scarce under the Empire due to the proliferation of *horti* and wealthy villas – and contributed to the complex pattern of activities on the margins of the city. Tombs and market-gardens were in competition for limited space, for example, and one solution commonly adopted was to surround a tomb with a productive smallholding (Purcell 1987: 35–6). Rome's markets occupied a pivotal position, excluded from the ceremonial centre but as close as possible to the capital's wealthy households and readily accessible from the farms which produced the goods it sold.

Wiseman has eloquently demonstrated the juxtaposition of 'luxury and poverty, beauty and squalor, love and death' on the Esquiline (Wiseman 1998: 22), and much the same was true of approaches to the city from other directions, that along the Via Appia in particular. For the last mile or so the grand monuments of the republican elite and the imperial house lay cheek-by-jowl with districts or buildings with much more mundane associations. Close to the Porta Capena lay the Area Carruces, where those leaving Rome could hire or load carriages (Rodriguez Almeida 1993c); nearby was the Area Radicaria, which was either a vegetable market or a complex concerned with the collection of customs dues on foodstuffs (Rodriguez Almeida 1993b). Flocks of sheep and goats waited for the attentions of the customs officers outside the city gates, before being led to the stock markets or *macella*. Wagons loaded with building materials trundled through the gates in long lines (Juvenal 3.255–61, with Delaine 1995: 558–9). Numerous bath-buildings are known to have been located in *regio I*, for example the balnea Abascanti, Antiochani, Bolani, Mamertini and Torquati; most of them must have been close to the Porta Capena and would have served the crowds of tired and dusty travellers as they entered the city. In imperial times the ancient grove of the Camenae outside the Porta Capena was notorious for the beggars who congregated there (Juvenal 3.15–16: see Rodriguez Almeida 1993d), seeking to accost visitors arriving in the city as well as exploiting the opportunities for scavenging and casual labour offered by the Area Carruces and Area Radicaria. Tombs around the city were used as houses by the desperately poor (*Digest* 47.12.3.11; Scobie 1986: 402–3), or occupied by prostitutes (Martial 1.34, with Howell 1980: 181; Martial 3.93.14–15; Juvenal 6.O.15–16); fear of witches, werewolves and the undead – all of which were thought to haunt cemeteries – would terrorise the passer-by (Horace, *Epodes* 5; *Satires* 1.8; Tibullus 1.5.53; Petronius, *Satyricon* 61–2; see Hope, in this volume). The whole area would have been shrouded in a dense pall of smoke from funeral pyres and from the furnaces of the baths (Robinson 1992: 116). Despite attempts by the elite at ostentation and display here, the poor and marginalised of Rome were so numerous and pervasive as to subvert attempts at grandeur.

Acknowledgements

I am very grateful to Roy Gibson, Keith Hopkins, Anneliese Parkin and Greg Woolf for helpful suggestions; also to the editors, the anonymous reader, and to Peter Garnsey for comments on earlier drafts of the paper. Those errors which remain are my own responsibility.

9

CONTEMPT AND RESPECT

The treatment of the corpse in ancient Rome

Valerie M. Hope

Introduction

The human body is something to be admired, pampered, neglected, abused and controlled either by the self or by others. Bodies and body parts are also loaded with cultural symbolism (Synnott 1993: 1). In ancient Rome, as elsewhere, not only did the body help to define essential identities such as those based on gender and age, but the presentation of the body through aspects such as dress, adornment and gesture could further codify the individual. Appearance could evoke respect, sympathy or revulsion. The toga was the prerogative of the citizen, the wearing of the purple distinguished the upper orders, while brands and tattoos indicated a criminal or servile past (Jones 1987; Sebesta 1997; Montserrat 1998). Public presentation and self-image were crucial aspects of how the identity of the living was both constructed and perceived. This processing was not immediately curtailed by death. A dead body could also retain a sense of self and identity. Yet as an inanimate object the corpse could become a powerful symbol, which could be honoured and prized or dismissed and despised by others. In simple terms, the distinctions of life could pervade death, and the treatment meted out to the corpse could parallel aspects of the life of the dead. The corpse could be used to reinforce or celebrate the identity of both the deceased and the survivors. Alternatively, the identity of the dead was open to manipulation, abuse and even destruction at the hands of others. As Parker has put it, 'Treatment of corpses remained one of the means by which men could hurt, humiliate or honour one another, express contempt or respect' (Parker 1983: 46).

Here I intend to examine the powers and symbolism attached to the remains of the dead. In short, how and why was the corpse honoured or dishonoured? Most of the subject-matter is drawn from the city of Rome, but where appropriate this is complemented by evidence from other parts of the empire. The time-span broadly covers the late Republic to the second century AD. In general, due to fundamental changes in belief concerning the soul and the body, early Christian evidence is excluded. The intention is to gain an overview of how the corpse was treated, regarded and exploited during the Roman period, but it should be noted that the available evidence often records the unusual and exceptional rather than the commonplace, and frequently reflects a public and male-dominated domain; hence the focus upon public honour and dishonour. The emphasis falls not on funerals and rituals, which are dealt with elsewhere in this volume, but on how and where the bodies of certain social groups were disposed of and how the physical remains, graves and memories of these same people were commemorated or obliterated.

Ensuring burial

Death creates a mixture of emotions and responses among the survivors. Love and affection or indeed fear or loathing of a person do not end with death. Death may also create new emotions of anger, guilt and remorse which are directed at the corpse (Grainger 1998: 38–41). These coupled with the ideas of decay, disease and pollution inherent in the body, and the fact that the body acts as a symbol of the mortality of the survivors, means that the dead are often treated with ambivalence. The corpse evokes both fear and solicitude, opposing views which are overcome by the observance of appropriate rituals (Malinowski 1925; cf. Frazer 1934–6). In Rome, as elsewhere, the ideal was that the dead should be treated with respect and properly disposed of. The dead were separated from the living by a series of rituals which fulfilled emotional, spiritual and practical considerations. It was important to do the right thing by the deceased in order to send the soul on its journey to the next world, to placate restless spirits, to remove a potential source of infection and to reintegrate the survivors into the world of the living. But the appropriate disposal of the corpse also sprung from a sense of human compassion and humanity. As Ulpian said, burial was a *negotium humanitatis* (*Digest* 11.7.14.7).

Descriptions of how the body was prepared for burial and of funeral rituals are limited and inevitably tend to focus upon the public and most striking elements. The unusual or the flamboyant, such as the embalming of Nero's mistress Poppaea or a grand funerary procession of a noble, might gain passing mention whereas more mundane details were little noticed (Tac. *Ann.* 16.5; Polyb. *Hist.* 6.53–4). To reconstruct the events surrounding death and burial often involves creating a patchwork picture from different types of sources, representing different places and times (Lindsay, in this volume). The evidence also provides few insights into the practicalities of disposing of the dead such as the role of undertakers and the expenses involved. Both inhuming and cremating a dead body can involve considerable amounts of labour and energy. Yet the digging of graves and the construction and tending of funeral pyres are little commented upon in the ancient sources (Noy forthcoming). This is not to say that disposal had to be expensive or elaborate. The most basic requirement was that the corpse should be covered with earth or in the case of cremation that a fraction of it was removed, prior to incineration, for later burial (Cic. *Leg.* 2.22.57). But people aspired to more than just the basics, and the efficient disposal of the dead, even if executed on a modest scale, probably represented a considerable cost to the bereaved family, heirs and survivors.

Failure adequately to dispose of the dead brought repercussions for both the living and the dead. Stories of wandering spirits and ghosts were often associated with incomplete or inadequate observance of burial rituals (Felton 1999: 9–12). The spirits of those who died violent or premature deaths might also be restless, especially if this was compounded by lack of burial (Virgil *Aen.* 6.320–85; Paus. 1.32.3–4; Tert. *De anim.* 56). The younger Pliny tells the tale of a haunted house the ghost of which was placated when its remains were discovered and given proper burial (*Ep.* 7.27). The ghost of the assassinated emperor Caligula was thought to haunt the area where he had been hastily cremated and buried until his remains were properly laid to rest (Suet. *Calig.* 59). The extent to which people actually believed in ghosts, spirits and the existence of an afterlife is unclear, but tales that told of the discontented dead reinforced the ideal that the corpse should be treated with respect (Bernstein 1993: 92–102). This respect probably had as much to do with the emotion, affection and duty felt by the survivors as religious sentiment. In *Aeneid*, Book Ten, as Aeneas slays Tarquitus he emphasises that his mother will never fulfil her duty by burying her son (10.557–60). Equally, the relatives and servants of traitors often sought to retrieve their mutilated bodies and afford them some sort of decent burial (see below).

The fate of the body could be a practical as much as a spiritual or emotional concern. No one wanted their remains, or the remains of their loved ones, to rot in public and to be a cause of offence to the living. The majority of people probably relied upon their nearest and dearest to do the decent thing without dictating specific requirements. Champlin has noted that in general testators were little interested with the precise details of their funeral and burial; they assumed that their heir would do what was appropriate (Champlin 1991: 170–1). By comparison, more testators devoted attention to their tombs; wills contained details about where the tomb should be built, how much money should be spent and how quickly the project should be completed (Champlin 1991: 172–5). The emphasis falls less on the fate of the bones and ashes of the deceased and more upon memory. The practical issue of burial coupled with the desire to preserve memory could also be addressed by the construction of a tomb before death. Many Latin epitaphs refer to such ante-mortem actions which were one way of choosing a suitable burial plot and ensuring that the commemorative epitaph and tomb matched expectations. That it could be better to do things for oneself is well illustrated by the tomb of Verginius Rufus, which ten years after his death was still unfinished (Plin. *Ep.* 6.10). Yet even if the tomb was completed before death the deceased was still dependent on others to perform the final rites, and to place the inhumed or cremated remains at rest in the chosen location. The tomb may have been made, a portrait commissioned and the epitaph cut, but did the remains always find their way to the right spot? A tombstone from Chester depicts and records a legionary centurion who was commemorated by his wife. The latter was pictured next to her husband and left a blank space underneath the portrait for the cutting of a second epitaph (*RIB* 491). This space was never filled. It is probable that the wife moved away or remarried and thus the tombstone became redundant. But we cannot completely dismiss the possibility that at death her wishes were overlooked or ignored. In Pompeii, Gaius Munatius Faustus built a tomb for himself and his dependants near the Nocera Gate (D'Ambrosio and De Caro 1983: 9ES). Yet it is doubtful whether his remains were ever interred here since his wife, Naevoleia Tyche, set up a second tomb at the Herculaneum Gate for herself and her now deceased husband. This tomb was a grand affair which drew heavily in its decorative schemes upon her husband's achievements but gave Naevoleia Tyche's name priority in the epitaph (Kockel 1983: 100–8).

For those without a pre-built tomb or property to bequeath by will the *collegium* offered a more modest alternative. While alive these societies provided their members, who were often connected by a trade, craft, religion or shared work in a large *familia*, with communal and social settings and could tie people to wealthy patrons (Patterson 1992). In death the regular payments made by the member facilitated burial. How many people belonged to *collegia*, built their own tombs or left instructions by will eludes us. But these strategies all involved preparing for death, primarily in financial and practical terms, but probably also to some extent emotionally and spiritually. Many others may not have confronted their mortality, either through financial disability or on the assumption that family and heirs would do the decent thing.

The living could make plans and express preferences about their burial and commemoration, but ultimately they had little control over the fate of their body. The dead put their trust in the living, and in most cases human decency, affection and religious scruples ensured that this trust was respected. Nevertheless, the law did provide a helping hand. In legal terms burying the dead was a financial priority for the survivors. It was best for the dead to be buried at their own expense, and this expense was more important than the receipt of legacies (*Digest* 11.7.14.1–13). Even when the estate was insolvent, funeral costs took precedence over all debts (*Digest* 11.7.45). Disputes could still arise as to who should pay for funerals and as to who was eligible to claim money from the estate for funeral expenses (*Digest* 11.7.14). But whether organised and paid for by the deceased or by the survivors, the ideal was for adequate disposal associated with appropriate rituals and commemoration.

The Roman funeral and cemetery undoubtedly reflected social aspirations and expectations. How the corpse was treated, buried and commemorated was one way that the living could negotiate status and reflect or construct desired identities. The normative rites were something to be adopted, adapted, elaborated, exaggerated or denied. In particular for those who existed at the extremes of honour and disgrace the means of life and/or the means of death could have dramatic consequences for the subsequent treatment of their corpses.

Honouring the honourable

The culmination of a successful public life was an honourable death followed by a suitable funeral and commemoration. Polybius provides a detailed account of a noble funeral of the Republican era. The corpse was at the centre of a series of events which aimed to honour the memory of the deceased. The body was paraded through the streets and then brought to the forum, the political and social hub of the city. Here the corpse was displayed on the rostra, and was sometimes even propped up, while a eulogy was delivered by a male relative. The listening crowd included people dressed up as and wearing masks (*imagines*) of the deceased's ancestors (Polyb. *Hist.* 6.53–4). The ceremonial marked the passing of the individual and simultaneously emphasised the continuity of the family both past and present and affirmed the rights of his heirs and successors. Polybius also emphasises that the whole populace could become involved in the funeral so that the loss of the deceased came to affect not just the mourners but everyone. The ideal was that the noble dead earned this honourable culmination to their life, and the praise and grief of the general populace, through a distinguished public career. Cicero emphasised that those who served the state were rewarded in life and also in heaven, where they would live among the gods (*Tusc.* 1.31.76). The final and ultimate earthly reward was a funeral and burial funded at public expense, an honour which was not attested before the time of Sulla (Flower 1996: 96). Cicero revealed some of the details and procedures for this in his proposal that Servius Sulpicius Rufus should be honoured not only with a bronze statue on the rostra, but also with a public funeral and the gift of a burial space which should be 30 feet in all directions (*Phil.* 9.7.16). Clearly a public tomb, as compared to the more normal publicly funded statue, would be a greater honour.

Under the empire the tradition of great aristocratic funerals continued and some of these may have been publicly funded (Tac. *Ann.* 4.13.6.27; *Hist.* 4.47). But the most elaborate funerary events involved members of the imperial family. These imperial funerals drew upon traditional aristocratic elements and involved processions, eulogies and the display of *imagines* (Price 1987). Extensive honours could mark the deaths of cherished members of the emperor's household. The heirs of Tiberius, Germanicus and

Drusus, were honoured in multiple ways which included the erection of statues and arches, the addition of their names to sacred hymns and the carrying of their images in public processions (Tac. *Ann.* 2.82.4.9). But the greatest posthumous rewards were reserved for the emperors, or at least those emperors who died honourably having designated a suitable heir. The funerals of these emperors were like pageants of Roman history and also incorporated elements of triumphal processions (Flower 1996: 107–9). The funerals to be sure were based upon Republican prototypes, but everything was writ large and the spectacle could culminate in the *apotheosis*, or the ascent to divinity, of the emperor. The funeral of the emperor was an opportunity for a great public display, not just of mourning, but of support towards and within the regime. Not only was the dead emperor honoured, but the new emperor asserted his power and celebrated his relationship with, in particular, the senatorial elite (Price 1987: 82–3).

The funeral was one part of the commemorative process which gave the corpse centre stage. Once the corpse was disposed of a monument could mark and protect the site of the grave, whether it contained cremated or inhumed remains. Compared to the transient funeral, a tomb could preserve honour and achievements in a more tangible and lasting form. This was true of any building or statue funded by or dedicated to the individual; but only in the tomb was the monumental complemented by both the physical and spiritual presence of the dead. At the death of the emperor both the tomb and *ustrinum* acquired a special reverence due to their associations with divinity. The first emperor Augustus created a large dynastic tomb on the Campus Martius, an area that lay beyond the *pomerium* or sacred boundary, but held a civic importance in the life of the city. Furthermore, this tomb was a grand statement about both the emperor and the system he was creating. Its sheer scale, visibility and environs made it a landmark in the city even if it lay technically beyond the walls (Zanker 1988: 72–7; Panciera 1994; Favro 1996: 117–19). The emperor Hadrian no doubt aspired to similar ambitions when constructing his tomb which drew heavily, in terms of its design and its integration into the city-scape, upon its Augustan precursor (Boatwright 1987: 165–81). In addition to the imperial tombs, the *ustrinum* or place of cremation, and the location of the *apotheosis*, could be marked and monumentalised. For Augustus the site of the *ustrinum* became a final but integral part of a series of related features and structures upon the Campus Martius that glorified the emperor and his regime (Boatwright 1985; Favro 1996: 170).

Public funerals, burials and commemoration also found their parallel in the cities of the empire. Those who had served their communities well might receive a funeral and a monument paid for out of public funds. This was often noted in the inscriptions that adorned funerary memorials. The epitaph of Aulus Umbricius Scaurus, a *duovir* from Pompeii, recorded how he was honoured by the erection of an equestrian statue in the forum and with a public funeral and monument at the Herculaneum Gate cemetery (Kockel 1983: 70–5). As a further distinction the graves of the distinguished might be placed close to, or within, the area known as the *pomerium*. This sacred strip which surrounded the walls of a settlement marked the area in which no bodies could be buried unless special permission was granted (Patterson, in this volume). In the necropoleis of Pompeii, graves were built in prime locations adjacent to the town gates and within the *pomerium*. The *augustalis* Marcus Cerrinius Restitutus was given a burial place, by decree of the decurions, close to the Herculaneum Gate (Kockel 1983: 47–51). Nearby was the grave of the priestess Mamia, which had also been decreed by the decurions (Kockel 1983: 57–9). The tomb of Mamia took the form of a semicircular seating area; a style of monument which had high prestige associations in the town (Kockel 1983: 18–22). In life these people had been prominent within the city; in death they were given prominent positions outside the walls. Life and death, inner city and outer city complement each other. At the heart of the settlement were buildings and statues honouring the achievements and gifts of leading citizens, while at the edge of the settlement were funerary monuments which also honoured this public role.

The cemetery like the forum could become an area for public and competitive display. The successful and wealthy could expect their corpses to be treated with respect, their lives honoured with grand funerals and their memories kept alive by suitable monuments. Yet the cemetery did not always reflect and promote the social hierarchy. It was only one possible arena for public display, the interest in which could rise and fall. Some questioned the relevance of funerals and monuments. Frontinus argued that a monument was a waste of money; a man would be remembered if his life deserved it (Plin. *Ep.* 9.19). For others the cemetery offered opportunities for ceremonial display that were rarely available in the centre of town. In death the epitaphs, statues and tombs of the cemetery could meet individual requirements and match an individual's own sense of pride and honour. But the details of monuments and concerns about their suitability were only relevant for those with sufficient money to make choices. For some even decent burial was a luxury.

Burying the poor

At the other extreme of society people left no lasting mark or reminder of their life. Some had no one to honour them or even to provide the most basic of funeral rites and burial. Unwanted bodies were left unclaimed or were deliberately dumped; corpses could be left to rot or were inadequately cremated or buried. At times of conflict and civil war the bodies of dead soldiers might lie unburied, slowly decomposing on the battlefield (Suet. *Vitell.* 10; Tac. *Hist.* 2.45). But even in times of relative peace and stability the disposal of corpses could present a problem within the urban environment.

Bodies or body parts could be a hazard for the living and an attraction to scavenging animals. Nero's escape from Rome was impeded by his horse becoming distressed at the stench of a rotting corpse (Suet. *Nero* 48). A human hand was dropped by a dog at the feet of the future emperor Vespasian, thereby prophesying his greatness (Suet. *Vesp.* 5). The body of an astrologer was cremated by Domitian to disprove the man's prophesy about his fate. But the corpse fell half burned from the pyre and was mauled by dogs, fulfilling the astrologer's predictions (Suet. *Dom.* 15). Martial tells of a dying homeless man who hears dogs howling in anticipation of his death and who is forced to flap his clothes to keep away the birds of prey (Mart. 10.5 10–12).

In Rome and elsewhere signs existed encouraging people not to dump rubbish, including corpses, within certain areas beyond the walls (*CIL* I^2 838, 839, 2981). To leave a body unburied offended religious scruples and moral ideals, but it was also a practical problem, an unsightly and unhygienic nuisance (Bodel 1994: 36–8). Evidence from Puteoli indicates that it was one of the roles of the public undertakers to gather up unwanted bodies and ensure that they were properly disposed of (*AE* 1971, n. 88; Gardner and Wiedemann 1991: n. 22). It is difficult to know just how many people had no one to provide for or care for their bodies. Bodel has estimated that for Rome as much as 5 per cent of the population may have fallen into this category and that perhaps as many as 1,500 corpses a year had to be disposed of at public expense (Bodel 1994: 41–2; and in this volume). These bodies may have been placed into mass communal graves. Varro explains that the pits into which the bodies of the poor were thrown were called *puticuli* (Varro *Ling.* 5, 25). Horace conjures up an evocative image of the pauper's burial ground on the Esquiline, where the corpses of slaves were carried on cheap biers and where whitening bones lay on the ground surface (*Sat.* 1.8.8–22). At the end of the nineteenth century Lanciani excavated, on the Esquiline, large man-made pits full of putrid remains including human bones which he believed represented the communal *puticuli* (Lanciani 1888; Hopkins 1983: 208–9; Bodel 1994: 40). The exact nature and location within the Esquiline of the *puticuli* remains uncertain, however, as does the fate of the bodies of the poor after the reclamation of the Esquiline under Augustus. Once cremation became the norm there may have been large-scale cremations of the bodies of the unwanted (Bodel 1994: 83); although Kyle has argued that the cost would have rendered this prohibitive and that burial within large communal graves continued (Kyle 1998: 169–70; cf. Bodel in this volume).

Approximately 100 years after Horace's description of the pauper's graveyard, Martial could conjure up a similar image of slaves carrying a body to the common graveyard where it would share the fate of thousands of others (Mart. 8.75.9–10). The end of the poor, the indigent and the abandoned was an anonymous and impersonal one. The unwanted dead were removed from the public gaze, but kindness, respect and honour were not the characteristics of the pauper's grave. This meagre treatment was a continuation of the misfortunes of life. For others the fate of their corpses reflected life's misfortunes, or a change in fortunes, even more dramatically.

Abusing the corpse

The sins of life could become the sins of the dead. Some individuals were excluded from full and proper burial procedures and further their bodies could be deliberately mutilated. In ancient Rome punishments were often designed to fit the crime, but they could also reflect the social status of the perpetrator. Those of high status might be offered an honourable exit – exile or death, either at their own hands, or rapidly and discretely by a swordsman (Bauman 1996: 124–8). For the less fortunate there was a myriad of awful deaths; crucifixion, burning alive and being thrown to the beasts. Humanitarian concerns about speedy and discrete executions are very much a modern invention (Coleman 1990: 461). Death became a public spectacle, and for the crimes of life, living bodies, and then dead corpses, were marked and mutilated, mauled and scarred and finally dumped.

Death itself did not always mark the end of the spectacle. Dead bodies, both in the flesh and pictorially, attracted the attention of the living. Images of fatal arena combats, victims at the point of death and wounded bodies were found in the domestic environment, especially in mosaics (Brown 1992). But the real thing could also become an object of display. For some, violent death was not the end of indignity; display of the corpse and post-mortem insults could form part of a punishment. The bodies of the crucified, for example, could be left upon the cross to rot. Following the revolt of Spartacus, 6,000 captives were crucified along the via Appia, from Capua to Rome, providing a potent image of the suffering and degradation that awaited those who dared to challenge authority (App. *B. Civ.* 1.120). In Petronius the crucified bodies of thieves from Ephesus were guarded by soldiers to prevent their removal (Petr. *Sat.* 111). Many executions took place at the edge of settlements and therefore near the cemetery zones. The contrast between the graves of the respectable on the one hand and the exposed rotting corpses of the damned on the other must have been a striking one (Kyle 1998: 53). The public dishonouring of the corpse could affect the elite and the once-powerful as much as the common criminal. Those accused of treachery or the losers in power struggles could expect little respect for their corpses. Their bodies might be displayed, not at the edge of the city, but at its very heart. Again the symbolism of contrasting fortunes must have been striking and also ironic for the onlookers. Once these victims had held sway and had been honoured at the centre of the city now they were displayed in disgrace at that same centre.

Under the empire traitors' bodies might be cast upon the Gemonian Steps or Stairs of Mourning (*Scalae Gemoniae*). Valerius Maximus states that these steps were in full view of the forum (6.9.13; cf. Richardson 1992: 345). References to the steps first appear in accounts of Tiberius' reign. The bodies of the emperor's many victims, including Sejanus and his children, were exposed here (Suet. *Tib.* 61; Tac. *Ann.* 5.10; Dio Cass. 58.11, 1–6). Tacitus and Suetonius both record that after Agrippina had starved herself to death, Tiberius claimed credit for not having her strangled and thrown onto the Steps of Mourning (Suet. Tib. 53; Tac. *Ann.* 6.24). An alternative, or addition to corpse exposure, was the dragging of the corpse, often by a hook, through the streets of Rome. Tacitus states that the rotting bodies of the supporters of Sejanus were dragged to the Tiber, while relatives and friends were forbidden to mourn or bury them (Tac. *Ann.* 6.16). The emperor Vitellius was tortured and executed, and then his body was dragged to the Tiber (Suet. *Vitell.* 17). The corpse of Elagabulus was dragged through the streets and even around the circus before being disposed of (*SHA Heliogab.* 17.1–3). The sense of irony in the public abuse of the corpses of the famous fallen is captured by Dio in his description of the demise of Sejanus. This man whom the crowd had previously escorted and courted was dragged to prison like the worst sort of criminal. The statues of Sejanus were toppled and destroyed paralleling the fate of his actual body. After his execution his corpse was thrown down the Stairs of Mourning where it was abused by the rabble for three days before it was thrown into the river (Dio Cass. 58.11, 1–6).

In a reversal of the role of the living body the corpse could become a passive object over which others had complete control. Possession of the body and mutilation of the body became the prerogative of the victor. Just as an emperor might legitimate his position by honourably burying his predecessor he could also legitimate his power by mutilating the corpses of his opponents or enemies. This was apparent in Tiberius' treatment of his family members. Augustus, his step-father and predecessor, was buried with all honours and ceremony whereas his great nephews and step-grandsons (the sons of Germanicus) were exiled and then either executed or forced to commit suicide before their bodies were chopped to pieces (Suet. *Tib.* 54). Similarly, Nero buried Claudius with due honour, even if Seneca quipped that he was dragged from heaven by the neck (Sen. *Apocol.* 11). Whereas Britannicus was buried hastily and without ceremony (Suet. *Nero* 33) and Octavia was exiled, killed and her head cut off for Poppaea to see (Tac. *Ann.* 14.61).

Decapitation of the corpse was a common act of mutilation. The heads of enemies and opponents were sought after and in some circumstances actively hunted down (Voisin 1984). With its easily recognisable features the head was particularly suited to display and abuse. In 87 BC the consul Octavius was killed by the forces of Cinna and Marius. According to Appian his was the first head of a consul to be displayed on the rostra in the forum (App. *B. Civ.* 1.71). Many heads were to share a similar fate, as a few examples will illustrate. In the proscriptions of 43 BC rewards were offered for the heads of the proscribed. Cicero's head and left hand were displayed on the rostra for a long time (Plut. *Ant* 20.2; Plut. *Cic.* 48.4–49.2). Octavian had the head of Brutus sent to Rome, where it was thrown at the feet of Caesar's statue (Suet. *Aug.* 13). The emperor Galba was decapitated by a soldier who unceremoniously presented the head to Otho with his thumb thrust into the mouth. Otho handed it over to some of his followers who stuck it on a spear and paraded it scornfully around the camp. This was not the end of the indignity since the head was sold to a freedman, whose master had been killed by Galba. This freedman promptly dashed his purchase to the ground (Suet. *Galba* 20; Plut. *Galba* 28.2–3). Galba's heir, Piso, was also decapitated, and Tacitus notes how Otho studied Piso's severed head with a particular malevolence (Tac. *Hist.* 1.44). The head could become a trophy for the victor. Its display almost served as a parody to the display of the *imagines* at elite funerals. The defeated lost the right to an honourable burial and rather than being accompanied to the grave by the facial images (*imagines*) of their dead ancestors their own contorted faces publicly announced their passing. This displaying of victims' bodies, and especially heads, had a particular potency when sovereignty was questioned or in dispute.

The mutilation of the corpse, and often its denial of burial, were part of a deliberate destruction of the identity of the deceased. Post-mortem sanctions and acts of *damnatio memoriae*, which could accompany public disgrace, had a similar effect. The individual had his property confiscated, his monuments destroyed and his name outlawed. Mourning for his death was limited and his *imago* or personal image, which would have been placed with those of the ancestors, was destroyed (Mustakallio 1994; Flower 1996: 23–31). The intention was to remove the identity of the accused, and during the Republic part of this process could also involve the levelling of the houses of those suspected of aiming at tyranny (Saller 1994: 93). The destruction and ransacking of houses could also be a ploy of political and military rivals (Cic. *Dom.* 108; Tac. *Hist.* 3.84). Could the houses of the dead, whether familial or individual structures, become the target for destruction and abuse in a similar fashion? Evidence from other times and places suggests that the graves and tombs of the dead can be at risk from the enemies of the living; the dead are vulnerable, and one way of insulting the religious and familial sensibilities of the living is through attacking the dead (e.g. Strocchia 1992: 33). The tombs of Rome's enemies were regarded as having no religious significance; material from them could be reused with impunity (*Digest* 47.12.4). By contrast, to despoil a Roman corpse or violate a grave was a capital offence. Sulla desecrated the grave of Marius, digging up the body and scattering the remains in the Anio river (Plin. *NH* 7.1.87; Cic. *Leg.* 2.22.56–7). Grave disturbance will be discussed further below, but in general political enemies do not appear to have followed Sulla's example and abused the corpse after it was interred. Cremation, which rapidly removed the individual features of the dead, may have reduced the vulnerability of the corpse, if not of the tomb structure itself. Prior to the anecdote about

Sulla, Pliny states that one of the reasons for the shift to cremation was that the inhumed bodies of men killed in distant wars were being disinterred (*NH* 7.1.87). Sulla himself, perhaps all too aware of what he had done to others, left strict instructions for his own cremation and burial. Others followed his example; one way of ensuring that the corpse would be spared disturbance and mutilation was rapid disposal. The body of Caligula was hastily cremated and buried, probably to prevent it falling into inconsiderate hands if recognised (Suet. *Calig.* 59; Noy forthcoming). Nero, horrified to hear that if executed his body might be dishonoured, started to prepare his own grave and made his companions promise that they would not allow his head to be cut off (Suet. *Nero* 49). Otho shared the same fear of decapitation and controlled the fate of his body by committing suicide and ordering his prompt cremation (Suet. *Otho* 10–11; Tac. *Hist.* 2.49). Vitellius would later visit the grave of Otho – but despite mocking its simplicity he did not violate or vandalise it in any way (Suet. *Vit.* 10).

Concerns about the fate of the body are a common preoccupation of those facing immediate and unavoidable death. The body is perceived to preserve identity even after life is extinguished. Whatever the nature of religious belief, there is a frequent shared desire to protect the body. For example, condemned prisoners in eighteenth-century England wanted above all else a decent and Christian burial rather than to fall prey to the knife of the anatomists (Gatrell 1994: 86–9). Such fears reflect human helplessness; even the most powerful in life are dependent upon others to protect them against insults once dead. Indeed the bodies of those who did not die as criminals, traitors or as the victims of civil discord could sometimes face insults. The funeral of the unpopular Pompeius Strabo, the father of Pompey, was disrupted by people dragging the body from the bier before officials intervened (Plut. *Pomp.* 1.2; Vell. Pat. 2.21.4). The emperor Tiberius died a relatively peaceful and aged death, but such was his unpopularity that the crowd rejoiced and threatened to drag his body by the hook, to expose it on the Gemonian Steps, to half-burn him and throw him in the Tiber (Suet. *Tib.* 75; cf. the threats made towards the body of Commodus, *SHA Comm.* 18.3–20.5). These threats paralleled the treatment that many others had received during the reign. But as always the new emperor had power over the body of the old emperor, and even Caligula would not dishonour a relative from whom he had derived his power and position.

The mutilation of the corpse was part of the extreme penalty paid by those who transgressed the laws. The prospect of this inspired fear and shame. But it only had a validity as a punishment because the destruction of the corpse broke all the normal and accepted taboos, values and behaviour. Even the pauper could hope to receive some sort of grave and to enter it whole. Not so the traitor and the criminal, whose deaths alone did not suffice; instead the state sought to destroy all aspects of their identity.

Denying burial

The final insult was not corpse mutilation but the denial of burial. Those left to rot on the Gemonian Steps or upon the cross received no final rites, no funeral, no burial, no tomb and thus no rest for their souls. They were cast out from the community and marked unworthy of burial; the best that they and their families could hope for was that eventually the body would be cast into the Tiber. Kyle has emphasised how it was the river of the city which probably acted as the most convenient and appropriate method of disposal both for the lowly criminals (*noxii*) killed in the arena and for the broken bodies of traitors. Kyle catalogues numerous examples of bodies that were dragged through the streets by a hook and then thrown into the Tiber (Kyle 1998: 218–24). 'The Tiber was the final stage in an elaborate ritual of abuse and vengeance, denial and damnation, a ritual familiar to plebeians, senators and emperors' (Kyle 1998: 222). The river washed away the remains of the enemies of the state and in the process purified the city.

Those facing death at treacherous times feared not just mutilation but that their bodies would never be buried. For Nero and Otho, whose plans were noted above, guaranteeing burial, preferably whole, was a prime motive for their suicide. Once more the right to grant or deny burial was the prerogative of the powerful and the victorious. To deny burial was the ultimate sanction and the ultimate display of power. Yet when this was taken to extreme, when the basic human right was repeatedly denied, the powerful left themselves open to criticism. In Tiberius' reign of terror the unburied body became an all-too-frequent sight. Tacitus uses images of heaps of bodies, rotting corpses and the inability of people to cremate, mourn or touch their dead to evoke sympathy (*Ann.* 6.17). On the other hand the victorious could place themselves in a good light if they did grant burial to the broken remains of their enemies. In fact such mercy could act as a more potent symbol of victory and power than denial. The body of Nero was allowed a decent cremation, burial and monument by a freedman of Galba's (Suet. *Nero* 49–50). Thus an ex-slave decided the final fate of the once most powerful man in the world. Even the heavily abused body and head of Galba (see above) were finally reunited and buried in his own tomb (Suet. *Galba* 20). Otho did not insist that the body of his opponent was dumped in the Tiber. Perhaps the most striking example is the treatment of Antony and Cleopatra by Octavian. The lovers were buried together, and Octavian ordered that the mausoleum they had begun in Alexandria should be completed (Suet. *Aug.* 17). The symbolism was explicit: the mausoleum stood for their failed attempt at power and their eastern leanings. By contrast the mausoleum of Augustus, constructed in Rome, celebrated his power and supremacy at the heart of the empire.

Denial of burial, however, affected not just criminals, traitors and the defeated. Others stigmatised by their profession may also have found themselves excluded from full burial rites. Their bodies may not have been mutilated or cast into the Tiber, but they may have been refused burial alongside their fellow citizens and the best they could hope for was the ignominy of the pauper's grave. A *senaltus consultum* from Larinum of AD 19 suggests that *auctorati* (contract gladiators) of high status were denied burial (Levick 1983). The meaning of the relevant part of the inscription is admittedly obscure, but Kyle argues that 'elite Romans who debased themselves in the arena might end up unburied' (Kyle 1998: 161). Those who willingly fought as gladiators are also singled out in an inscription from Sarsina, probably dating to the first century BC, in which a Horatius Balbus donated burial plots for the town's inhabitants (*CIL* XI 6528 = *ILS* 7846). *Auctorati*, although not specifically those of high status, were excluded from burial in these plots. The implication here is that although not all gladiators were denied burial, some were.

This treatment of the gladiator relates to the degrading nature of the profession, but also the ambivalence it engendered. The gladiator was a skilled combatant, a champion of the arena and a popular hero, yet he was stigmatised by his lowly status, by the exploitation of his body for entertainment and by the blood that he spilled (Wiedemann 1992: 26–47, 102–24; Barton 1993). The gladiator was simultaneously honoured and dishonoured, and this could continue after death. Unlike the criminal killed in the arena, the gladiator was given the opportunity to fight for his life and even gain his freedom. If killed in combat the corpse of the gladiator might receive reasonably decent treatment compared to the *noxii*. Surviving tombstones and epitaphs suggest that the bodies of at least some gladiators were claimed and received burial in a marked grave (Hope 1998; Hope forthcoming). The sense of comradeship and the existence of *collegia* may have all helped the gladiator to avoid non-burial and the *puticuli*. This is not to deny that many gladiatorial corpses may have remained unclaimed and were disposed of unceremoniously. Even for those gladiators who did receive decent burial, their graves may have continued to bear the marks of their disgrace and *infamia*. Gladiators may have been allowed access to the cemetery only grudgingly; it is possible that their graves may have been grouped together, apart from others, or close to the amphitheatre in which they had died (Hope 1998). Their identity in life defined their identity in death, they were marginalised to the last. This said, it appears that only *auctorati*, those free men who willingly became gladiators, could actually be denied burial altogether, and for this practice the evidence is very limited. In some circumstances it would appear that these men, especially those of high status who broke all the accepted codes, paid for this not only by their violent death, but also by their loss of burial.

The inscription of Horatius Balbus also denied burial in the donated land to those who hanged themselves or who followed some immoral trade for profit. Like the gladiatorial profession, other activities marked the participants with *infamia*, which entailed legal and social disadvantages. Undertakers, actors, pimps and prostitutes were among the stigmatised. They sold and degraded themselves for others or were polluted by activities which others shunned (Gardner 1993: 128–53; Edwards 1997). Actors like gladiators could earn fame, fortune and following, and surviving tombstones suggest that they could be decently buried and appropriately commemorated (*ILS* 5180–5276). How prostitutes, undertakers and others faired is unclear. Some may have prospered, but many would have been slaves, ex-slaves and non-citizens who like other elements of the urban poor struggled in life and received little recognition in death. In many ways this underclass occupied an underworld which has left little trace. This is especially ironic for those employed in undertaking roles, such as corpse-bearers, and also for prostitutes, since these figures haunted the cemetery in life (see below; and also Bodel and Lindsay in this volume) but left little trace there in death.

For others it was not the activities and crimes of life that earned them non-burial but the means of death itself. Horatius Balbus singled out those who hanged themselves. The exclusion of suicides from the cemetery and normative rites would fit with other times and places. Although fundamental changes in belief, especially due to Christianity, need to be gauged, suicides have often been regarded as transgressing accepted boundaries. In Tudor and Stuart England, for example, suicide was a crime, and suicides were tried as self-murderers, their property was confiscated and their bodies were denied Christian burial. Until the early nineteenth century English suicides could be buried at a crossroads with a stake driven through their hearts (Macdonald and Murphy 1990: 15–41). An element of softening English attitudes towards suicide originated in elite interests in Latin literature, since the suicide of noble figures such as Cato came to be viewed as a model for the gentlemanly exit (Macdonald and Murphy 1990: 179–82). Indeed in the ancient world suicide was viewed with some ambiguity. Some forms of suicide and reasons for committing suicide were honourable, and suicides were not, in general, denied burial. A handful of epitaphs even appear to record the fact that the grave belonged to one who had chosen their own time and means of death (Van Hooff 1990: 151). Historical accounts are peppered with descriptions of the suicides of those for whom it was politically expedient to end their days. Tacitus notes that for some who stood accused of treason, specifically during the reign of Tiberius, suicide was a way not only of avoiding the executioner, but also of ensuring that their property remained intact and that their body was properly buried (*Ann.* 6.21). Suicide could also serve as a method for making a statement about or criticism of the existing political regime; although all such acts were not simply gestures of freedom, since if allowed or encouraged by the emperor the suicide could become a symbol of the emperor's power (Plass 1995). Nevertheless, many suicides were described in admiring detail. The emperor Otho, as noted above, accepted his defeat, and chose his own manner of death, thereby ensuring that his body would not be mutilated and would be buried properly. Tacitus and Suetonius both note that his grave was marked by a modest but lasting tombstone (Suet. *Vit.* 10; Tac. *Hist.* 2.49). Tacitus also described the suicide of Seneca. Under threat of the death sentence, Seneca took his life with great dignity. His cremation was without ceremony at his own instructions (*Ann.* 15.62). These suicides were performed in the face of death and represented an honourable exit and to a degree an assertion of political freedom (Plass 1995: 85); there was little question that the bodies of these self-killers should be in any way punished (Desideri 1995: 197–203).

Some suicides, their means and methods, however, did cause moral, social and spiritual issues for the living. Legal texts underline this, 'people do not go into mourning for those convicted of betrayal, nor of those who have hanged themselves and those who laid hands upon themselves, not because they were sick of life but from consciousness of guilt' (*Digest* 48.21.3.2). This does not suggest that suicides were left to rot, but in some circumstances the suicide could be equated to a criminal, an aspect of whose punishment could be exclusion from burial. Further, in popular belief the soul of the suicide was punished. Those who killed themselves were victims of a violent and unnatural death which might leave their spirits or souls trapped between the world of the living and that of the dead (Van Hoof 1990: 162–5). In the *Aeneid* Virgil has those who died at their own hands occupy a separate and discontented part of the Underworld (6.434). Artemidorus suggests that suicides were not named among the dead who were remembered by relatives at death meals (*Oneirocritica* 2.50). There was a possibility that if allowed burial in the cemetery the soul of the suicide would be a dangerous and threatening presence. Quintilian turned the question as to whether the self-killer should remain unburied into a rhetorical exercise. He argued that self-killing is not the same as killing another and that the body of the suicide does not deserve the same fate as the criminal (Quint. *Institutio Oratoria* 7.3.7). But in Lanuvium a funeral *collegium* specified that those who laid hands on themselves would not receive their burial allowance (*CIL* 14.2112; Hopkins 1983: 215). Perhaps this was to prevent abuse of the society's funds, but the stipulation may have had a spiritual dimension aiming to protect the communal burial space against the presence of restless souls (Van Hooff 1990: 116). In general, however, it was the means as much as the motive for suicide which could lead to the exclusion and dishonouring of suicides. Hanging, as singled out by Horatius Balbus and the *Digest* (see above), seemed to be an infamous and dishonourable exit. In Puteoli it was specified that the bodies of the hanged were to be removed by the public undertaker within an hour of their being reported (*AE* 1971 n. 88; Gardner and Wiedemann 1991: n. 22). Of all the ways to choose to die hanging was despised and the corpse of the culprit was punished, 'hanging distinguished a sissy from a man' (Van Hooff 1990: 67; Desideri 1995).

To deny burial was to contravene all the standard spiritual, moral and practical norms. It debarred the deceased and their family from what was expected in terms of affection, duty and human decency. Further in common belief denial of burial precluded the soul from moving on; it was trapped between this world and the next. The unburied were denied full access to the community of the dead. For some this paralleled the position they held in life; gladiators, for example, were kept on the margins of the community of the living and remained on the margins of the community of the dead. For others this denial was part of a whole process of punishment and retribution. It made clear that the dead were powerless, but that corpses could become powerful symbols in the hands of the living.

Interfering with the body

Some aspects of corpse abuse could have more sinister and secretive causes and motives. For some the bodies of the dead held a fascination or special powers which could render the body little more than a commodity. Once more it was the poor, the dishonoured and the disreputable who were probably most at risk. At one end of the spectrum was the use of bodies for scientific study. Human dissection was a taboo, and Pliny suggests that it was sinful to look at human entrails (Plin. *NH* 28.5). Nevertheless, both human dissection and vivisection were not unheard-of in antiquity, and during the Hellenistic period condemned criminals may have been utilised by doctors (Edelstein 1967). As in England, before the passing of the Anatomy Act, such dissections both furthered scientific knowledge and served as part of criminal punishment. For the Roman period there is little evidence for human dissection. Galen appears to have regretted this, although he implies that in Alexandria dissection might still occur (Gal. *De anatomicis administrationibus* 1). In general, the only option to study anatomy was through the dissection of animals; monkeys and apes being particularly useful. Galen's description of a group of physicians watching the dissection of an elephant and the removal of its heart suggests the importance of observation even if this procedure was executed by the imperial cooks (Gal. *De anatomicis administrationibus* 7.10). Indeed, human corpses, even if they could not be dissected, could be observed in various stages of decomposition. Galen describes how he had seen dead bodies after tombs became dilapidated and in one case because a flood washed a body out of its grave. The exposed bodies of criminals might also prove useful; Galen saw the skeleton of a robber which had been left to rot because no one wanted to bury it (Gal. *De anatomicis administrationibus* 1). So the bodies of the injured, the dying and the dead were a crucial source of information. But there was no ancient equivalent to the nineteenth-century resurrectionists who supplied anatomy schools (cf. Richardson 1988).

Bodies may not have been stolen in the name of science, but there is some evidence for bodies and body parts being procured, or at least sought after, for other purposes. Petronius tells the tale of a soldier posted to watch the bodies of the crucified. While he is distracted one of the bodies is removed by the deceased's family. The soldier makes use of a body from another grave to conceal his neglect of duty (Petron. *Sat.* 111–12). The body-snatching tale makes for an entertaining story, but if corpses did have any value it may have been motivated more often by superstitious beliefs. Pliny lists, with a hefty dose of scepticism, some of the cures which were reportedly to be obtained from corpses and body parts. The touch of the dead could cure a patient of the same sex, especially if the deceased had died prematurely; pills made from the skull of a hanged man were good for dog bites; sore gums could be cured by scraping them with a tooth of a man killed by violence; the hair of a man taken from the cross could also have beneficial properties (Pliny *NH* 28.7–45). The examples repeatedly suggest that violent and premature death imbued the dead with special powers. This is perhaps most graphically illustrated by the consumption of the leg-marrow and brains of infants and the suggestion that drinking blood from gladiatorial wounds could cure epilepsy (Pliny *NH* 28.4–5). For comparison, in eighteenth-century England superstition suggested that corpses of the hanged held therapeutic and healing properties. In Wessex it was thought that ulcers and cancerous growths could be cured if touched by the hand of an executed criminal. People might fight their way through crowds to the gallows to touch the dead. Yet such behaviour was not akin to corpse abuse or robbery since, instead of humiliating or abusing the corpse, it placed it in esteem (Linebaugh 1975: 109–11; Gatrell 1994: 81). Similarly in the Roman context those who were degraded, despised and feared could be elevated by the attainment of magical properties at death. In the case of the gladiator this once more underlined the ambivalence of his position; he was polluted by the blood that he spilled while his own blood and body were prized. Pliny's list, which aims to shock as much as inform, does not enlighten us as to how the relevant parts of the bodies of the dead were procured or touched. But the bodies of the unclaimed and the exposed bodies of criminals may have been particularly susceptible to those who sought souvenirs, amulets and cures.

The powers of the corpse might also be harnessed through curse tablets or *defixiones* which called upon the dead to perform a special task for the living. Many of these were placed in graves, and once more the graves of those who had died premature or violent deaths, whose souls were thought to be discontented and trapped between the world of the living and the dead, may have been targeted (Gager 1992: 18–20). Witches were also thought to frequent the graveyard, exploiting the dead and their remains. Horace describes witches on the Esquiline collecting bones and harmful herbs (*Sat.* 1.8.19; cf. *Epod.* 5). The witches of Thessaly were particularly notorious. Apuleius tells the story of a man visiting Thessaly who was asked to guard a corpse against body-snatching witches. These witches would gnaw the flesh off dead men's faces to use in their witchcraft. In this case, however, the guard was so effective that the witches removed his nose and ears rather than those of the corpse (Apul. *Met.* 2.21–30). Necromancy or raising the dead to predict the future was also allegedly practised in Thessaly. The man who guarded the corpse was only made aware of the loss of his own extremities when the corpse was briefly brought back to life to accuse the widow of committing murder. The most lurid description of necromancy is found in Lucan. The son of Pompey, on the eve of the battle of Pharsalus, seeks out the most famous of Thessalian witches, Erictho. This witch regularly steals the bodies of the dead from funerary processions, the pyre, sarcophagi, from the gallows and the cross. Lucan implies that she feasts off the dead, plucking out their eyeballs and gnawing on their nails. To tell the future for Pompey she uses the corpse of a recently killed soldier which is still lying on the battlefield. The corpse is dragged away by means of a hook and rope, and then the body is opened up. Blood and potions are poured into the body cavity, and with invocations to the gods, the dead man is brought back to life (Luc. *Pharsalia* 6.413–830; for further examples of necromancy see also Sen. *Oedipus* vv.530–626; Heliod. *Aeth.* 6.14–15).

Lucan's account is extremely fanciful, and is intended to shock the reader with a series of gruesome images, but it is not entirely impossible that he had heard of or witnessed experiments in such areas. The emperor Nero, whose court Lucan frequented, was fascinated by such ghoulish proceedings (Luck 1985: 192). Even if we dismiss the idea that witches regularly stole corpses, the possibility still existed in the popular imagination; and even if necromancy was never a reality, we should not doubt that the cemetery in general might become the focus of strange activities and that the corpse itself could become the focus of unwanted attentions.

Interfering with the grave

The efficient disposal of the dead protected the living by removing a spiritual, hygienic and practical problem. Simultaneously disposal also gave the dead protection from the living by preventing physical mutilation and spiritual or magical exploitation. Yet burial, whether of ashes or a corpse, did not necessarily mark the end of the living's interference with the dead. The boundaries between the living and the dead could be porous (Bernstein 1993: 84–106). This is well illustrated by beliefs that the dead were still present. Ghost stories, the powers attributed to the corpse and the annual festivals to remember and placate the dead suggest that, at least for some, the dead continued to have a shadowy, if ill-defined, existence (Felton 1999). The living and the dead interacted; their worlds were not clearly demarcated or separated. This interaction was reflected in the physical and practical organisation of the cemetery. The dead were removed from the living; they occupied their own settlement beyond the walls of the town. In many ways the cemetery was a marginal space: at the edges of life, concerns and activities (see below). But in acknowledging the marginal side of the cemetery we should not dismiss it as a completely dead and inactive space. The Roman cemetery was not clearly marked and defined. Tombs fronted the roads; they were visible and accessible; you did not have to make a special trip to the cemetery to be confronted by tombstones and epitaphs. Equally, the suburban area was not the preserve of the cemetery and the funerary monument. Villas, gardens and workshops could jostle for prime space outside the walls. The suburb, including the tombs, was in many respects an extension of the town rather than separate from it (Purcell 1987; Patterson in this volume).

The proximity of the living and the dead could lead to a conflict of interests. The grave was regarded as a sacred place which was not to be interfered with. Those accused of deliberately violating graves suffered *infamia*. Anyone who despoiled a corpse could endure the death penalty or the mines (*Digest* 47.12.3.7). Similarly those found guilty of removing or scattering bones could face the supreme penalty (*Digest* 47.12.11). In theory, once in the grave, the body and remains of the dead were safe. It was noted above how people were eager to secure rapid burial to avoid corpse abuse and denial of burial rites. There were, however, exceptions to this security; Sulla's desecration of the grave of Marius is the most notable example of a powerful individual carrying out what otherwise would be a heinous act. Others may not have gone to such lengths, but graves and their contents might still be disturbed for political and symbolic ends. Both Augustus and Caligula interfered with the grave of Alexander the Great. Augustus had the sarcophagus containing Alexander's mummy removed from its shrine and crowned the mummy with a golden diadem (Suet. *Aug.* 18); while Caligula wore a breast-plate he had stolen from the tomb (Suet. *Calig.* 52). These anecdotes served to illustrate Augustus' respect on the one hand and Caligula's disrespect on the other. But it was a sign of both their authorities that they had access to the tomb. Entering the mausoleum also emphasised the veneration for Alexander and the continuing potency of Alexander's identity which was enshrined in his remains. The political value of bodies could also increase when power changed hands. Suddenly those who had been rejected, and perhaps even denied burial, could become powerful symbols and reintegrated. Caligula made a great display of gathering up the bones and remains of his mother and brother, alleged victims of Tiberius, and reburying them with due honour (Suet. *Calig.* 17). This was the act of a dutiful son and brother, but it also helped to underline his connections with once popular figures. Bodies and graves could both acquire and lose political potency.

The graves of most people were not political and may not have attracted undue attention from either enemies or supporters. Yet even the most humble grave could be at risk from the living. The grave was sacred, but interference and even removal could sometimes be justified. The grave itself might contravene what was expected and acceptable. Domitian had a tomb destroyed, and the bones and ashes it contained thrown into the sea, because the founder, the son of an imperial freedman, had built the tomb with materials which were intended for a temple (Suet. *Dom.* 8). Graves built on public land could also cause problems. Cicero tells of a large-scale exhumation of graves from public land outside the Colline Gate (Cic. *Leg.* 2.23.58). Those who were buried in tombs or on land which did not belong to them, might also not rest in peace for long, although the actual owner of the property would need to gain permission from the pontiff or emperor before the offending remains could be removed (*Digest* 11.7.7–8). Legal debates about who owned graves, and rights of access to them, suggest that, as with all property, a grave could be at risk of unsympathetic use, resale and disrespect. No doubt tombs were demolished and the remains dispersed to suit the needs of changing times and changing generations even if this was not always strictly legal. At the very least the ideal was that the actual physical remains of the dead should be treated with respect. The construction of the basilica over tombs in the so-called Vatican necropolis, despite or perhaps because of changing religious times and sentiments, appears to have been executed with some sympathy for both the dead and their families. Some remains may have been removed to new sites, and the tombs themselves were not demolished (Toynbee and Ward-Perkins 1956: 12–13). Sacral law did allow graves to be moved if they became dangerous or were threatened by flood (Robinson 1975: 183). In short, despite their sacred and inviolable nature, cemeteries, tombs and individual graves could be moved or destroyed in response to the forces both of man and of nature.

The fact that people feared what would happen to both their tomb and their remains is often witnessed in surviving inscriptions. Epitaphs call for fines and curses against those who may interfere with their graves (Robinson 1975: 180–1). But rarely is it clear who will police such threats. Some surrounded their tombs with gardens, perhaps intending their heirs and successors to use any profit from produce for the upkeep of the tomb. Others made provisions in their wills for guardians to maintain and protect their resting-places (Champlin 1991: 176). Trimalchio planned to have a freedman stand guard over his tomb (Petron. *Sat.* 71). We can only speculate how long such measures were honoured and thus effective. The tombs and graves of earlier generations, and also the wishes and preferences of their inhabitants, were probably quickly forgotten. The bricks and mortar of a tomb might live on, and the epitaph might continue to promote a name, when there was no one left with actual memories of those commemorated or with any interest in respecting their wishes. The demands on and changes made to tombs and burial spaces are well illustrated by the Isola Sacra necropolis. Here the founders of the individual house-tombs tried to record in the titular epitaphs who would have access to the tomb, but their original intentions were often subverted. With time, spaces within the tombs were given or sold to others, tombs were subdivided or their internal organisation was disrupted by the introduction of inhumation burials (Hope 1997).

The graves of the dead were at risk from the living. Space outside the walls was often at a premium and, whatever the details of the law, the tomb was property to be bought and sold, bequeathed and divided up, cared for or neglected. But amongst all this activity we have to acknowledge that it was its very nature that made the cemetery vulnerable. Interaction between the living and the dead may have been substantial; the cemetery may have been of great symbolic importance, an extension of the town and at times even busy and bustling. Yet in many respects the cemetery remained a liminal space. Not only was it located on the edge of the settlement, but it was the home of the dead – who were gone yet still present. At night, in particular, the cemetery was a disquieting place, filled, in the popular imagination, with ghosts and wandering spirits; a place that attracted the low-life of the town. Cemeteries were the haunts of beggars, thieves, prostitutes and witches. Lucan's Erictho was said to live in abandoned tombs (Luc. *Phars.* 511–12); Horace has witches wandering the Esquiline (*Sat.* 1.8.19); Petronius sets the tale of a soldier who turns into a werewolf in a cemetery (Petron. *Sat.* 62); Martial refers to whores who haunt the cemetery and take cover in tombs (1.34.8, 3.93.15); Apuleius describes thieves using a tomb as a stash for their loot (*Met.* 4.18.21); legal texts suggest that the homeless might live in tombs or set up establishments there (*Digest* 47.12.3). Marginal activities were at home in a marginal zone. All this served to subvert the dignity of the cemetery and the respect that the dead deserved (cf. Patterson, in this volume). If the bones of the dead remained unearthed and undisturbed, and if their tombs were not sold, or divided or ransacked for building materials, the dead were left to share their homes with tramps and prostitutes.

Conclusion: resting in peace

The ultimate transition of and modification to the human body is death. The body changes from a living, breathing, moving state to become inanimate and decaying matter. How much of the identity and individuality of the living is preserved in the corpse and for how long is an issue for both the dying and the bereaved. In the Roman world there were a range of beliefs about the soul, its continuity, and the afterlife. But whatever the spiritual beliefs of the individual, the fate of the remains of the dead, the residues of their physical identity, had to be confronted and dealt with. Life is centred on defining, modifying and controlling the body. The final and absolute loss of control of the body was often feared since at death the body passed into the hands of others. The fate of the corpse, if not always the soul, was dependent on the living. The living controlled dead bodies.

The corpse could become a potent symbol which was open to abuse and manipulation. Who possessed the corpse, buried the corpse, commemorated the corpse and subsequently had access to it were crucial issues both within the family and wider power structures. In some respects the corpse could become a trophy to be honoured, displayed and paraded before it was finally disposed of. The dead through wills and pre-death planning might attempt to dictate the terms of their burial and commemoration, but ultimately the dead were powerless. In general the wishes and expectations of the deceased were probably fulfilled but there was always the risk of a range of insults, however minor. A miserly funeral or an inadequate monument could make a petty but effective final comment by ungrateful heirs. At the other extreme the enemies of the dead might abuse the corpse or desecrate the grave. The living always held the upper hand. Yet, in speaking of the relationship between the living and the dead in terms of power and control, there is perhaps a risk of losing sight of individuality and that every corpse was unique. In fact individuality was the very key to this process; to honour the corpse or to abuse it was tied to the preservation or destruction of individual identity.

Despite being physically powerless the corpse could become imbued with power. The bodies of the mighty, for example, could retain their potency. The physical remains and the tombs of people such as Alexander the Great or the emperor Augustus attracted the living and could help to define the identity of the living. To enter the tomb, to touch the remains or to claim the right to be buried alongside these figures was a source of power. The corpses and body parts of lesser mortals could also fascinate the living; doctors, witches or those searching for a cure might physically harm the body, but all, in their own way, elevated the dead and associated specific powers with the corpse. The powers associated with the body would perhaps be taken to their extreme in the Christian context, despite the associated changes in belief. The reburial of the remains of saints and martyrs in prime locations, the desire of the living to be buried in close proximity to them, and the search for relics, whether body parts or clothing, expressed honour for the corpse, while simultaneously leading to the desecration of graves and the destruction of physical remains (Clark 1998: 108–10).

The treatment of the corpse was one way of expressing contempt or respect for the life of the deceased; praise and blame continued beyond the point of death. But ambiguity often underpinned and even undermined these judgements. For emperors death might mark the first point when judgement might be passed. Tiberius and Claudius received decent burial by their successors, but not all agreed that this was deserved. The abuse of the bodies of traitors might evoke sympathy rather than revulsion. Even the bodies of criminals and gladiators could be elevated at death by gaining magical and curative powers. All this underlines the general ambivalence felt towards the dead. The corpse is and is not the person who once lived; the dead are gone but still present; memories are both prized and forgotten; the cemetery is both protected and neglected.

Here I have been primarily interested in the ways in which the corpse was idealised or demonised and how the corpse could become a powerful symbol in the negotiation of power and identity. This is not to deny the cathartic, emotional and religious content of funeral rituals and the commemoration of the dead. Death could trigger spiritual concerns about the fate of the soul, a sense of familial duty, practical concerns about disposal and a myriad of human emotions. These aspects were all bound up with the public symbolism and potency of the corpse and it is not always possible or desirable to separate the differing strands. How the corpse was finally treated, disposed of and commemorated was influenced by many factors which reflected the views, beliefs, feelings and requirements of both the dead and the survivors, whether the latter were only the immediate family or the wider populace. The treatment of the corpse, whether it was honoured or abused, was based upon the adherence to or denial of what was expected in terms of emotion and belief, honour and duty. In many ways this chapter has focused on the extremes of this behaviour; how the dead of the elite were honoured; how the dead of the poor were neglected; how the corpses of criminals and the defeated were abused; in short how the dead were exploited by the living. Much of the evidence reviewed has painted a bleak picture of the treatment of the corpse. The risks the dead faced from the living were manifold; a corpse could be abused, mutilated and denied burial; a grave could be desecrated, sold or destroyed. It was not just the corpses of the poor and the disgraced which were at risk; a tramp, a body-snatcher or a developer paid little respect to distinctions of honour and rank. All this suggests that for the dead, resting in peace was hard to achieve. Thus to end it is worth noting that the reality for the majority may have been somewhat different; a decent if modest burial, with no abuse or mutilation, in a grave undisturbed, if not always remembered, for centuries.

Acknowledgements

I would like to thank Janet Huskinson and David Noy for reading and commenting upon an earlier version of this chapter. Any errors, however, remain my own.

10

DEALING WITH THE DEAD

Undertakers, executioners and potter's fields in ancient Rome

John Bodel

Death-pollution for the Romans was a mixed thing, part religious concern, part practical problem. That is a truism applicable, no doubt, to most cultures, but it will serve to mark the two ends of a spectrum that embraces much of Roman mortuary ritual. The challenge for the student of Roman customs is to recognise where along the scale between those two poles any particular behaviour is to be located. This chapter attempts to chart three distinct positions by focusing on Roman attitudes toward the professionals responsible for conducting funerals and performing public executions and on Roman practices in disposing of the bodies of the least fortunate. As an avowedly preliminary excursion, it makes no pretence to comprehensiveness and intentionally steers clear of some important areas traditionally covered in discussions of Roman death-ritual – the cult of ancestors and *imagines*, for example, or the sanctity of tombs (Flower 1996; De Visscher 1963; Ducos 1995) – which have tended to focus almost exclusively on upper-class behaviours, in the hope that an approach to the problem from the bottom up, rather than from the top down, may offer a fresh perspective.

Potter's fields

> Here nauseous weeds each pile surround,
> And things obscene bestrew the ground:
> Skulls and bones in moulding fragments lie,
> All dreadful emblems of mortality.
>
> from Webb's *Collection of Epitaphs* (1775)
> (Wilson and Levy 1938: 16)

How many people died in Rome each year and how many, lacking formal burial arrangements, depended for the final disposition of their remains upon the services of the state? If we adopt a conservative estimate of the urban population around the time of Augustus of roughly 750,000 (cf. Hopkins 1978: 96–8; Robinson 1992: 8; Lo Cascio 1994: 39), and if we further postulate an annual mortality rate comparable to that of other pre-industrial European urban populations of roughly 40 per thousand (cf. Parkin 1992: 92; Saller 1994: 12), we must figure that some 30,000 residents died in the city each year, or (on average) more than eighty a day. In times of epidemic, of course, the numbers would have risen dramatically. We may doubt Jerome's claim that during a plague in AD 77 nearly 10,000 a day died at Rome over a period of several weeks (*Chron.* 2096I, p. 188h Helm), but Cassius Dio's figure of 2,000 a day succumbing during the outbreak of AD 189 sounds plausible (73.114). According to Suetonius, 30,000 urban residents died during one plague-ridden autumn under Nero (*Nero* 39.1; cf. Oros. 7.7.11; Shaw 1996:115–18). In European towns from the fourteenth to the seventeenth centuries, occasional outbreaks of the plague often carried off from a quarter to a third of a town's population in a single year (Mols 1954–6: 2.426–52; Biraben 1975: 1.192–218).

At all periods a few of those who died at the capital would have been buried elsewhere, at an ancestral grave on a country property or outside an Italian town, but these can never have amounted to more than perhaps one or two per cent of the urban population, probably considerably less. We must then figure that, over the three hundred years from 100 BC to AD 200, the cemeteries of Rome had to accommodate nearly nine million burials of one sort or another, whether cremations or inhumations. We must also suppose, even when due allowance is granted to the popularity of funerary *collegia* and the habit of some wealthy Romans of providing burial space for their slaves and freedmen in familial monuments (Patterson 1992; Eck 1988), that a certain number of urban residents living in abject poverty and without the support of a patron must have fallen through the cracks. When these hapless souls gave up the ghost, the disposition of their corpses became, for them, a source of anxiety, for others, at the very least, a problem of urban maintenance. Martial (10.5.9–12) imagines a dying beggar envying those borne off in a pauper's bier and dreading the predatory post-mortem attacks of dogs and birds. Such fears would not have been unfounded. In 276 BC wolves dragged a half-eaten corpse into the Forum (Oros. *Adv. pagan.* 7.4.1–2); closer to Martial's own day, the future emperor Vespasian was interrupted while dining by a dog that dropped a human hand beneath his table (Suet. *Vesp.* 5.5; cf. Cic. *Mil.* 33; Scobie 1986: 418–19). For Rome's poorest residents, the fate of their last remains was a legitimate concern; unlike most Romans, when they died their bodies were likely to wind up as *cadavera*, abandoned flesh, rather than *corpora*, corpses destined for burial (Allara 1995). What percentage of the urban population fell into this unfortunate category at any point in time is impossible to say, but a reasonable guess might place their number in the neighbourhood of one in twenty.[1] On a conservative estimate, then, some 1,500 corpses may have turned up annually, unclaimed and unwanted, in the streets of Rome.

Based, as they are, upon a number of unprovable hypotheses, any of these figures could be disputed, but some comparative data suggest that they are not likely to be far out of line. Even in modern cities, disposing of the corpses of the indigent presents a considerable practical problem. During the first half of 1994, for example, more than 150,000 persons died in Moscow, a metropolis of about nine million, and the demand for burial in or near the city surpassed 400 per day (Specter 1994). In New York City nearly 75,000 of the 7.3 million residents die each year, and more than 3,000 unclaimed bodies wind up annually in the public potter's field on Hart Island in the Bronx, a barren 101 acres that have provided a final resting-place for some 700,000 New Yorkers over the last 125 years (Conlan 1993: 42, 49–50). Rome itself during the nineteenth century – a period that saw the urban population grow from around 125,000 at the start of the century to more than 225,000 at its close – experienced between 4,000 and 6,000 deaths each year, except in times of epidemic, which were not infrequent, when the number rose to more than 12,000 (Forcella 1984: 291 n. 10). During the Great Plague of London of 1665, when the city population numbered somewhat under half a million, 68,596 succumbed to the disease, according to the Bills of Mortality, and the total is in fact likely to have approached 100,000 (Bell 1924: vi–vii, 123, 144–52; cf. Mols 1954–6: 2.442–4). If we extrapolate from those figures and allow for a slightly higher incidence of mortality within a larger urban population, we arrive at figures very close to those postulated for ancient Rome.[2]

There can be little doubt that the ancient Romans faced a significant challenge in their efforts to provide burial facilities capable of meeting the demand imposed by high mortality in a growing population. How they met this need during the late Republic is well known from a passage of Varro (*LL* 5.25), a poem of Horace (*Sat.* 1.8), and a fortuitous discovery made by Rodolfo Lanciani outside the Esquiline Gate more than a century ago (see below). None of these sources, however, says a word about the institutional mechanisms for removing unclaimed corpses from the urban centre. To get a sense of those we must turn to comparative evidence from ancient Athens, Egyptian Thebes, and Puteoli.

In fourth-century Athens the *demarchoi* were responsible for seeing that abandoned corpses were buried and the affected demes purified, if possible by the relatives of the deceased or, failing that, at public expense ([Demosth.] 43.57–8; cf. Arist. *Ath. Pol.* 50.2; *IG* II^2 1672.119–20). It is therefore a reasonable, if not absolutely necessary, inference that at Rome the removal of dead bodies from city streets was considered a part of the *cura urbis*, a charge that normally fell to the *aediles* (Mommsen 1887–8: II^2 505–17). According to the terms of a contract for the local funerary concession at Puteoli sometime toward the end of the Republic, persons who abandoned corpses there were fined, and the undertaker was obliged to remove the bodies of executed criminals, suicides by hanging, and slaves; this was the public service for which, in return, he was granted a monopoly concession (*AE* 1971, 88 I.32–II.1, II.13–14, II.22–3, III.1–4). It is perhaps unlikely that a single corporation of undertakers was responsible for policing the entire city of Rome, but there is no reason to think that the business of disposing of the dead was conducted there in any fundamentally different way, and the institutional imitation that characterises Puteoli's relationship with the capital points in the same direction (Bodel 1994: 15–16). In Egyptian Thebes of the Ptolemaic period, the city and surrounding territory were divided up among various morticians, who enjoyed exclusive rights to prepare for mummification the bodies of those who had resided in their allotted areas (*P. Tor. Amenothes* 5, 8; *UPZ* II p. 200; Derda 1991: 17–18). Perhaps a similar division of labour by district served the urban zone of Rome. It is in any case clear that, except in times of plague, when extraordinary and frequently inadequate measures were taken to dispose of diseased corpses in the Tiber and the public sewers (Dion. Hal. *Ant. Rom.* 10.53.2–3, 9.67.2; further Lugli 1952: II.46–51 nos. 264–96), the bodies of Rome's indigent, wherever found, wound up in the same place.

According to Varro, outside of Roman towns were *puticuli*, named from *putei*, because men used to be buried there in pits, or else, as his teacher Aelius Stilo had written, because the corpses abandoned there used to rot (*putescebant*) in a public place beyond the Esquiline (Varro *LL* 5.25). Varro goes on to add that the playwright Afranius jokingly called them *putilucos*, because the bodies there received light through the wells (*CRF* 430 Ribbeck), from which we may infer that the *puticuli* were normally left open to the skies, as was the normal practice in early modern Europe in Hamburg, Paris and England (Whaley 1981: 104; Ariès 1981: 56–9; McManners 1981: 304; Gittings 1984: 64). Varro's description seemed to be strikingly confirmed when, toward the end of the nineteenth century, construction of a new residential district on the Esquiline in Rome just outside and north of the Esquiline Gate laid bare some seventy-five mass burial pits, rectangular in shape, arranged in rows, lined with blocks of *sperone* or *cappellaccio tufa*, and set off from the surrounding cemetery by a travertine channel (Lanciani 1874, 1875, 1890: 64–5). These mass graves have naturally been associated with the public potter's field described by Horace in the last satire of his first book as a pestilential region 1,000 by 300 feet in area strewn with bones, which Maecenas sometime around 40 BC buried under his suburban *horti* (Hor. *Sat.* 1.8.8–16; cf. Häuber 1996). In fact, the burial vaults discovered by Lanciani cannot have been part of the paupers' cemetery described by Horace, since they seem to have been covered over by a layer of rubble and charred debris nearly half a century earlier, at a time when a section of the trench along the Servian *agger* just north of the Esquiline Gate had been filled to the brim with corpses (Bodel 1994: 38–54), and it has been denied that they are *puticuli* of the sort described by Varro (Coarelli 1999a). For the present purpose it is enough to note that the vaults uncovered by Lanciani are similar in size and shape to the mass graves employed for the burial of the poor in France and England from the sixteenth to the eighteenth century (see Table 10.1).[3]

The comparative evidence suggests that the Roman vaults might have contained between 550 and 800 human bodies each. In fact, Lanciani reports animal carcasses and other detritus mixed in with the human remains, so we cannot calculate an absolute burial capacity for the Roman pits; but the figures cited above provide suggestive enough indication that the crypts must have remained open for several weeks or even months before being filled to capacity – long enough, certainly, that putrefaction of their deposits would have begun to set in and the unpleasant symptoms of decay (stench and putrid air) would have emanated into the environs. In London during the Great Plague of 1665, a large mass burial pit (Table 10.1) was filled with more than 1,100 bodies within two weeks (6–20 September) during a time of exceptionally high mortality (Wilson and Levy 1938: 15); under normal circumstances rotting flesh was exposed to the environment for longer periods. In Paris one or two grave pits remained open for months or even years before being filled (Ariès 1981: 56), and the problem of putrid odours polluting the vicinity persisted well into the eighteenth century (McManners 1981: 308–9). There can be little doubt that when Maecenas buried the paupers' graveyard outside the Esquiline Gate at Rome under thirty feet of virgin soil he abated a significant public nuisance.

Table 10.1 Size and capacity of mass burial pits in London, Paris and ancient Rome

Dimensions (feet)	*Capacity (cubic feet)*	*Bodies*	*Cubic feet per corpse*	*Location (and date)*
15 × 40 × 20	12,000 [8,400]	1,114	[7.5]	London (1665)
15 × 18 × 30	8,100	1,200–1,500	[5.4–6.75 !]	Paris
15 × 18 × 20	5,400	600–700	[7.7–9.0]	Paris, Les Innocents (1763)
15 × 15 × 18	4,050	500	[8.1]	Paris, Rue de Bagneux (1746)
12 × 12 × 30	4,320	[540–575]	(7.5–8)	Rome, Lanciani's *puticuli*
13 × 16 × (30)	6,240	[780–830]	(7.5–8)	Rome, Lanciani's *puticuli*

Sources: London: Wilson and Levy 1938: 15; Paris: Ariès 1981: 56–8; Rome: Lanciani 1875: 43; 1890: 64; cf. 1874 'di varia grandezza'.

Note: Figures in square brackets are deduced; those in parentheses are hypothetical. The approximate capacity of the grave pit at London is based upon the datum that it was filled to within six feet of the surface with 1,114 bodies.

What end awaited the corpses of the poor after that time remains uncertain, but we do not hear further of mass burial pits and none from the early imperial period has been discovered. A decree of the senate of 38 BC, probably passed in conjunction with Maecenas' closing down of the potter's field on the Esquiline, forbade the burning of bodies within two miles of the city (Cass. Dio 48.43.3), and Porphyrion, commenting on Horace's satire, says that the Esquiline was made healthier because the crematoria (*ustrinae*) were moved farther away (Porph. ad Hor. *Sat.* 1.8.14); he says nothing of new *puticuli*.[4] In the preceding note (on *Sat.* 1.8.11), Porphyrion refers to public crematoria (*haec regio namque publicas ustrinas habebat*), but it is unclear whether at 1.8.14 he refers to public facilities rather than to private ones, or indeed whether his information is accurate: possibly he is merely connecting the senatorial decree reported by Dio with Maecenas' works. There is in any case reason to believe that Maecenas' closing of the Esquiline graveyard marked the end of the practice at Rome of burying the poor in mass graves and that subsequently cremation in public crematoria became the common fate of those without the means to ensure a private burial. When Lucan imagines the pauper's funeral that would suffice to honour Pompey, he speaks of placing the body on a humble pyre (8.736–8). Martial, in describing an encounter late at night in the streets of Rome with four tattooed corpse-bearers carrying out a pauper's cadaver, remarks that the unlucky pyre receives a thousand such (8.75.9–10). And when Plutarch mentions the practice among corpse-burners of stacking one female cadaver with every ten male bodies, since the fattier tissue of women helped to feed the flames, he is clearly thinking of mass crematoria (*Quaest. Conv.* 3.4.2 = *Mor.* 651B).

To anecdotal literary evidence of this sort it has been objected that references to pyres for the poor may be merely 'figurative' and not to be taken literally and that mass crematoria would have been impractical because of the risk of fires and the difficulty of creating sufficient heat to reduce human corpses to ash and bone (Kyle 1998: 169–70). But ancient pyres were fully capable of sustaining temperatures as high as 900 degrees centigrade, the average achieved by modern crematory furnaces (Wells 1960: 35–6), and a Roman cremation of a single corpse could probably have been completed within seven or eight hours (McKinley 1989: 65). Indeed, large communal pyres such as that mentioned by Plutarch would have burned hotter and faster, once fully ignited, than individual specimens. As for the risk of fires, this was no doubt real, but precautions had been taken by the senate already in 38 BC, and at Ostia, where practices were probably not dissimilar from those at Rome, individual tombs with their own *ustrinae* built on the rear and lined with heat-resistant bricks were in common use just outside the city beginning in the first half of the first century AD (Floriani Squarciapino 1956: Via Ostiensis no. 20a/b, Via Laurentina nos 32, 34, 43, etc.). In fact, it is precisely during the Augustan era that monumental *columbaria* designed to accommodate the ashes of multiple cremations begin to appear along the Via Labicana-Praenestina outside the Esquiline Gate (Häuber 1990: 15, 65), and there is reason to see the Augustan period as marking a decisive turning-point in Roman funerary behaviour, with public attention shifting from the traditional focus on the cortège through the city streets and funeral oration in the Forum to the extra-mural grave-site and the pyre (Bodel 1999: 270–6). It seems reasonable to conclude that at Rome under the early Empire, mass cremation replaced mass burial in grave-pits as the preferred means of disposal of the bodies of the indigent.[5]

Nowhere are we told of any reason for this change. The silence of our literary sources is perhaps not surprising, but the absence of any hint of religious or ethical concerns about the treatment of the corpses of the poor marks a notable contrast with public perceptions in early modern Europe of the horror of a pauper's funeral (e.g. Laquer 1983; Gittings 1984: 64, 67). If we are right in associating this change of custom at Rome with the closing down of the Esquiline potter's field by Maecenas and the enactment of new legislation forbidding the burning of bodies within two miles of the city, it is plausible to suppose that a primary motivation was simply a concern for the public good. Whether or not the specifically sanitary dangers of decomposing corpses were recognised, the sights and smells of rotting flesh had evidently grown offensive by Horace's day, and the layer of charred debris strewn across the mass grave pits unearthed by Lanciani suggests that the risk of fires from crematoria in the region was real (Lanciani 1874: 52; cf. Bodel 1994: 45–7).

There is no sign in any of this of a Roman concern with religious pollution. On the contrary, in their arrangements for the disposal of the bodies of the needy, the Romans seem to have been motivated by purely pragmatic concerns. In contrast to the sanctity of tombs, which were regarded as *loca religiosa* (Ducos 1995; De Visscher 1963: 43–63), the suburban areas set aside for the disposal of the indigent were not accorded the status of graves but were instead classified as *loca publica*, places owned by the *populus Romanus* and designated for the use of all (Mommsen 1895: 207–8 [202–3]). Unlike tombs, these public spaces could not be encumbered with private religious observances (Cic. *Leg.* 2.58); conversely, *loca religiosa* could not be declassified and treated as profane (*Cod. Iust.* 3.44.9 [Phil.]). To judge from a passage of Papinian's monograph on the upkeep of cities in which the abandonment of cadavers is listed beside dumping dung, brawling, and discarding animal skins in a list of acts prohibited in town streets, this secularisation of the disposal areas of the indigent extended to the treatment of their corpses as well (*Dig.* 11.7.43.2a). Roman authorities evidently treated the problem of disposing of unclaimed corpses as a simple matter of public policing rather than as a cause for concern about religious pollution. In this respect, Roman custom differed sharply from the practice at Athens, where, as we have seen (above, p. 130), the *demarchoi* were responsible not only for removing abandoned corpses but also for ritually purifying the infected demes.

Undertakers

Death is bad for those who die but good for the undertakers and grave-diggers.
(*Dissoi Logoi* 1.3)

When we turn to Roman attitudes toward the professionals who actually handled corpses, from places to personnel, we encounter a more ambivalent situation. As mediators between the worlds of the living and the dead, undertakers and other workers in the funerary trade are the human agents of the institutional mechanisms societies create in order to accommodate both the public need to ensure the efficient disposal of human remains and the nearly universal desire on the part of the living for respectful treatment of the dead – to bridge, in other words, the gap created by that fundamental human polarity Malinowski describes as 'love of the dead and loathing of the corpse' (Malinowski 1954: 47–8). Undertakers thus represent a natural focal point of a complex of values that are often themselves inherently contradictory: their work is generally regarded as both necessary and distasteful, as at once purifying and inherently sordid.

Some societies respond to this paradox by constructing occupational hierarchies that distance the diverse mortuary specialists from the rest of the community according to the degree of their involvement with the corpse. So, for example, among contemporary rural Cantonese, funerary workers are shunned in proportion to their exposure to the pollution of death: geomancers, who divine the appropriate locations for tombs and have no direct contact with the dead, rank at the top; corpse handlers occupy the bottom and are pariahs in the community (Watson 1982, 1988; Lindsay, in this volume). The same sort of hierarchy is found in contemporary Hindu society (Parry 1980). Similarly, in Egypt of the Ptolemaic and early Roman periods, *taricheutai*, or 'embalmers', enjoyed the privileges of priests, whereas the morticians who actually prepared the corpses for embalming, the *paraschistai*, literally 'the ones who rip up lengthwise', were treated as scapegoats: once they had slit open the corpse with the ritually prescribed 'Egyptian stone' (probably flint), they were driven from the scene under a hail of stones and curses aimed at directing divine retribution for violating the body onto their own heads (Diod. Sic. 1.91.4–5; cf. *UPZ* 194–6). The former were regarded as ritually pure, the latter as permanently defiled (Derda 1991: 15–21).[6]

In Rome, on the other hand, we find no such sharp distinctions among the various specialists. Already by the time of Augustus, it seems, workers in the funerary trade were grouped together and were regarded similarly. So much, at any rate, is suggested by the use under the early Empire of the vague and euphemistic terms *Libitina* and *libitinarius* in reference to the business of undertaking. The former is first attested in the so-called Julian law on municipalities inscribed at Heraclea in Lucania shortly after Caesar's death (*CIL* I^2 593 = *ILS* 6085 = *FIRA* 1 no. 13 = Crawford 1996: 1 no. 24, 94–6, cf. 104–7), where the phrase *libitinam facere* is used to describe the activity of undertaking, the latter in a ruling attributed to the Augustan jurist Labeo, who holds a *libitinarius* liable for a theft committed by his slave mortician (*Dig.* 14.3.5.8). The earliest literary attestations belong to the age of Nero (Petr. 38.15, 78.6; Sen. *Ben.* 6.38.4). *Libitinarii* seem to have been funeral contractors and suppliers of workmen rather than tradesmen themselves, but their name betrays their close association with the specialist personnel under their supervision. The designation 'one associated with Libitina' does not, however, take us very far, since the term 'Libitina' enjoyed a remarkably broad semantic range in popular usage of the early Empire.

The word appears metaphorically for death itself, as in Horace's famous boast at the end of his first three books of *Odes* that a large part of him will avoid Libitina (3.30.7); or, by metonymy, for the apparatus of burial, as in Martial's expressions 'one Libitina will carry out two (corpses)', where 'Libitina' evidently stands for 'bier' (Mart. 8.43.3–4; cf. Plin. *NH* 36.45; *CGL* VI.1.641–2), or 'Libitina is being piled up with papyrus ready to burn', where 'Libitina' means 'pyre' (Mart. 10.97.1); or more vaguely for funerary facilities generally, as in a proverbial phrase twice employed by Livy to describe the exigencies faced by early Romans in times of plague, when 'Libitina was insufficient for the number of funerals' (40.19.4, 41.21.6); or for burial itself, as in a decree of the Roman senate of AD 19 from Larinum, in which those found guilty of having practised disgraceful professions are prohibited 'from having Libitina' (*AE* 1978, 145, line 15; cf. Bodel 1994: 98 n. 69); or even for the actual business of undertaking, as in the phrases *libitinam facere* (*Tab. Heracl.* [*CIL* I^2 593 = Crawford 1996: 1 no. 24] lines 94, 104–5) and *libitinam exercere* (Val. Max. 5.2.10; *lex Puteolana* [*AE* 1971, 88] II.16–17, III.20–1), which were the standard ways to describe the activity in the early Empire.

Plutarch (*Numa* 12.1) identifies Libitina as the goddess of funerals, but in placing her among the deities of the underworld he is probably mistaken, since there is no sign that Libitina ever entered the Roman pantheon. As far as we can tell, she had no temple, no cult and no worshippers (Thaniel 1973: 48–9). Primarily this morbid figure is associated with a grove at Rome (cf. *CIL* I^2 1268, 1292, 1411; a *pagus Libitinus* is attested at Ligures Baebiani: *CIL* IX.1455 = *ILS* 6509 add. [III.54]), and her 'name' *libitina* or *lubentina* was probably in origin no more than a toponym related to Etruscan *lupu* or *lupuce* (= *mortuus est*) (Freyburger 1995: 215–16; cf. Walde and Hoffman 1938: 1.794; Ernout and Meillet 1959:

355–6). Romans of the late Republic derived her name from *libido*, 'sexual pleasure', and associated her with Venus – naturally since there was a temple of Venus located in her grove (Varro *LL* 6.47; Cic. *Nat. D.* 2.61; cf. Non. Marcell. p. 89.16–17 L.; August. *De Civ. D.* 4.8). According to the annalist L. Calpurnius Piso, King Servius Tullius, wishing to know the population of the city, ordered that a coin be paid for each death 'into the treasury of Venus in the Grove, whom they call Libitina' (ap. Dion. Hal. *Ant. Rom.* 4.15.5); and Festus tells us that a temple to Venus was dedicated *in luco Libitinensi* (he uses an adjectival form) on August 19, the day of the 'Rustic Vinalia' festival (Festus 322 L.; cf. Paulus 323 L.). T. P. Wiseman has recently coaxed out the implications of Festus' notice to illuminate the associations of this hybrid Venus Lubentina, as guardian of gardens, with Venus Erycina, patroness of prostitutes, at the Colline Gate, whose cult was celebrated on the other day of the Vinalia festival, April 23 (Wiseman 1998). The topographical juxtaposition of the two Venuses at either end of the Servian *agger* helps to confirm the location of the Grove of Libitina outside the Esquiline Gate, in the region of Lanciani's *puticuli* and Horace's potter's field, and perhaps points to a popular association of the pleasures of the flesh associated with Venus Erycina and the inevitable end of all mortal flesh so vividly evident in the vicinity of Venus Libitina. Artemidorus comments on the case of a man who, having dreamed he had entered a house of prostitution and was unable to leave, died a few days later: 'it is reasonable that this place should resemble death, because a whore-house is known as a common place (*koinos topos*), like that which receives corpses, and much sperm perishes there' (Artemid. 1.78 p. 87.33). The connection between sex and death was commonplace in antiquity; less well attested is this apparent conceptual association of 'low', unproductive, sex with 'low', unfulfilling, burial, of brothels and potter's fields.

However that may be, Plutarch tells us that 'things for burial' (*ta pros tas tafas*) were sold in Libitina's precinct (Plut. *Quaest. Rom.* 23 = *Mor.* 269A–B), and although he does not specify precisely what apparatus is meant, we may surmise that it included such essential equipment as funeral beds (*tori Libitinae*, [Quint.] *Decl. Mai.* 9.6) and biers (Varro *LL* 5.35, 166), torches (e.g. Mart. 8.43.2), incense and perfumes (Mart. 10.97.2; Pliny *Epist.* 5.16.6), and perhaps the clothes in which the deceased was dressed for burial (*vitalia*, Sen. *Epist.* 99.22; Petr. 77.7–78.1). From a comment of Asconius we learn that the *fasces* traditionally borne by lictors at the head of the cortège of an aristocratic funeral were kept at the grove of Libitina (*In Milon.* 34). No doubt Plutarch's 'things for burial' included not only funerary equipment but funerary services. The pseudo-Acro scholia on Horace in any case inform us, explicitly if not entirely authoritatively, that Libitina was the place in the city where those who contracted to carry bodies out for burial and who provided 'what was necessary for funerals' (*funeribus necessaria*, cf. Sen. *Ben.* 6.38.1) were located ([Acro] ad Hor. *Sat.* 2.6.19). We need not follow Piso in believing that the presence of Libitina at Rome went back to the regal period, but her grove is attested as early as 166 BC, and there is no difficulty in believing that from any early date workers in the funerary trade made their headquarters in the region of the public cemetery where they performed much of their work. Later, during the middle and late Empire, mortuary workers were known collectively as *funerarii* (e.g. Firm. Mat. 1.135.21, 1.168.20, 2.349.8; cf. Derda 1991: 35 for a similar development from the Ptolemaic to the later Roman period among funerary workers in Egypt). Earlier we hear only of various specialists designated by their individual names.

Our earliest references, in Plautus, are to *pollinctores*, morticians, who took their name from the practice of covering the face of the corpse with powder (*pollen*) in order to conceal the discolouration of death (Plaut. *Poen.* 63; *Asin.* 910; Var. *Men.* 222, 324; *Dig.* 14.3.5.8 [Labeo]; Mart. 10.97.2; etc.; cf. [Serv.] ad *Aen.* 9.485). We hear also of *vespillones*, corpse-carriers, so called, according to Festus, not because of any connection with wasps (*vespae*), but because they carried out in the evening (*vespertino tempore*) the bodies of those without the means to afford a proper funeral (Paul. exc. Fest. 368–9; cf. [Serv.] ad *Aen.* 11.143); a modern etymology relates the name to *versipellis*, 'werewolf': as an attacker of humans, a despoiler of corpses, a werewolf is *vespiliator* (Knobloch 1991). Whatever the origin of their name, these pall-bearers of the poor were evidently a recognised presence in Roman life already by the middle years of the second century BC: so we may infer from the report that the aedile Q. Lucretius in 133 ordered the body of Tiberius Gracchus to be cast into the Tiber and thus earned for himself the scarcely honorific *cognomen* Vespillo (*De Vir. Ill.* 64.8; cf. Val. Max. 1.4.2; Kajanto 1965: 324). Other sources mention *fossores*, 'grave-diggers' (*CIL* VI 7543, 9655), and *ustores*, 'corpse-burners' (Cic. *Mil.* 33; Catull. 59.5), as well as flautists (*tibicines*: Cic. *Leg.* 2.59; Paul. exc. Fest. p. 982 L.) and special horn players (*siticines*, *tubicines*: Cato *Orat.* 220 [= *ORF*^{4} 8.223, pp. 90–1]; Nonius p. 54), mimes and dancers (Dion. Hal. 7.72; Suet. *Caes.* 84; *Vesp.* 19; Appian *Lib.* 66) and lictors (Cic. *Leg.* 2.61). From the earliest days of the Republic, hired women dirge-singers, *praeficae*, sang the praises of a dead man in front of his house – a custom especially remarked by Aristotle in his treatise on the 'Customs of Foreign Peoples' (cf. Varro *LL* 7.70; Non. Marc. 66.27; Kierdorf 1980: 94–105); according to the grammarian M. Aurelius Cotta they came from the Grove of Libitina (Funaioli *Gramm. Rom. Frag.* 90). Festus records a shrine of the goddess Nenia ('Dirge') outside the Viminal Gate (Festus p. 157 L.), halfway between Venus Libitina outside the Esquiline Gate and Venus Erycina outside the Colline Gate, at the other end of the Servian rampart. Perhaps this shrine to Nenia marked the northern boundary of the area outside the Servian *agger* in which the various funerary tradesmen were headquartered, an area bounded on the south by the Grove of Libitina, where, it has been argued, the flute players' guild was located (*CIL* VI 3877 = I^2 989; cf. Bodel 1994: 50).

Consolidation of the various specialists of the funerary industry at Rome in a single location may have fostered among them a certain community of interest and, on one occasion, at least, moved them to act in concert: Valerius Maximus reports that in 43 BC, when a decree of the senate authorised the praetor to hire out the contract for undertaking the funerals of the two deceased consuls, Hirtius and Pansa, at public expense, 'those who practised undertaking promised both their equipment and their services free of charge ... and furthermore extracted the concession that the job of providing the apparatus for the funeral cortège be awarded to them for a single sesterce' (5.2.10). The task of arranging the cortège normally fell to a funeral director known as a *dissignator*, whose status may have been somewhat higher than that of the other tradesmen (e.g. Hor. *Epist.* 1.7.6; Sen. *Ben.* 6.38.4; [Quint.] *Decl. Mai.* 6.8). The title was often associated with that of *praeco*, 'herald' or 'auctioneer', whose position in society, though far from elevated, seems to have been less despised than that of those who handled corpses directly (Hinard 1976: 740–6). Certain Romans of the late Republic and early Empire, at any rate, were not ashamed to proclaim themselves as both *praecones* and *dissignatores* on their tombstones – something that cannot be said of *libitinarii* or other workers in the funerary trade (*CIL* I^2 2997a [p. 971], X 5429, perhaps XI 4596). The distinction probably arises from the degree of specialisation associated with the several professions: whereas *libitinarii* were exclusively involved with funerals and the dead, *praecones* and *dissignatores* practised their trades in other areas of public and private life as well – in making announcements and auctioning property (*praecones*: Mommsen 1887–8: I^3 363–4) or in serving as ushers at the theatre (*dissignatores*: Plaut. *Poen.* 19–20; *CIL* VI 1074, VIII 32332) or, beginning in the Hadrianic period, as referees or umpires at athletic contests (*Dig.* 3.2.4.1). In the case of the *dissignatores*, the role of usher may have grown out of that of funeral director, inasmuch as the task of arranging seats at the scenic games traditionally held in conjunction with aristocratic funerals would naturally have fallen to the man charged with organising the funeral parade (for which see Flower 1996: 97–106; Bodel 1999: 263–5); that of referee perhaps arose from a transfer of the authority inherent in one who assigns seats to spectators to that of one who adjudicates priority in athletic competition.

However that may be, uncertainties about the connection between undertakers (or ushers) and auctioneers (or heralds) centre on a clause of the *Tabula Heracleensis* prohibiting 'those who practise auctioneering, funeral directing or undertaking' from seeking, accepting or holding political office in the community, so long as they practise those professions (*CIL* I^2 593 = *ILS* 6085 = *FIRA* 1 no. 13 = Crawford 1996: 1.24, 94–6).[7] We need not here enter into the long history of the discussion of this vexed passage (Lo Cascio 1975–6 provides a clear exposition of the issues); for our purpose it is enough to consider a recent argument that the restrictions imposed upon these three occupations have nothing to do with their association with death (Gardner 1993: 130–4). Gardner rightly points out that religious dread played little part in Roman civic regulations regarding the disposal of the dead and concludes that the prohibitions in the *Tabula Heracleensis* arose instead from the lawmakers' desire to avert a potential conflict of interest in municipal officials, in that auctioneers, funeral directors and undertakers 'did paid work for the local authority' (Gardner 1993: 134; similarly already Nicolet 1966: 1.403–4, accepted by Crawford, in Crawford 1996: 1.384). Explicit evidence that any of these professionals was paid to perform public work, however, is difficult to find, and the one specific instance adduced of a supposed conflict of interest points to the opposite conclusion. According to the terms of the *lex libitinaria Puteolana* (*AE* 1971, 88), the contracting undertaker, in addition to his other duties, was obliged to perform public executions at a magistrate's bidding; this assignment, it is supposed, might potentially have influenced a contractor sitting on the town council to line his pockets by voting unduly readily in favour of punishments. But at Puteoli the law explicitly requires the contractor to perform public executions free of charge (*gratis praest(are) d(ebeto)*: *AE* 1971, 88 II.11–14); this was the return given to the community for the award of a lucrative public contract. Nor is it clear, if conflict of interest were the primary issue at Heraclea, why the law prohibits practising heralds, funeral directors and undertakers not only from holding but even from standing for public office: in mere candidates, no conflict of interest could arise. The specificity of the *Tabula Heracleensis* on this point, as well as on the types of occupation censured, is to be noted: at Halaesa in Sicily anyone who had ever practised a profession was excluded from local office (Cic. *II Verr.* 2.122; cf. Lo Cascio 1975–6: 364–6).

Gardner rightly notes that auctioneers, like undertakers and funeral directors, 'were unpopular because they reminded people of things they would prefer not to think about' but misses the significance of Cicero's remark to the effect that witnessing the enforced sale at auction of one's own property is like attending one's own funeral, when buyers come not as mourners but as executioners to pick apart the corpse (*Quinct.* 49–50). It is not simply that death and bankruptcy were unpleasant to think about but that both involved an unwilling transfer of property, without compensation. The stigma attached to the professions of auctioneer, funeral director and undertaker – and to workers in the funerary trade more generally – arose principally, I suggest, from the perception that their livelihood came at the cost of another's loss. The well-known paradox of Roman attitudes toward money-making is that while the accumulation of wealth was perfectly respectable and having more of it than your neighbour was generally a good thing, profits should never come at another's expense. Cicero in a famous passage of *De Officiis* provides the classic statement of Greco-Roman aristocratic disdain for hired labour in general and for occupations that generated public animosity in particular (1.150–1; cf. Brunt 1973). The undertaking profession falls into both categories, as Roman authors repeatedly emphasise. Seneca refers to a lawsuit won by Demades against a mortician at Athens on the grounds that he had hoped for great profits and could only have attained his wish by the deaths of many; the philosopher goes on to remark that legacy-hunters are like undertakers and funeral directors, only worse, since the latter pray only for anonymous deaths (*Ben.* 6.38.1, 4). The salient point is that undertakers were supposed to be venal and malevolent; hence the frequent allusions in literature of the early Empire to deaths as Libitina's profit (e.g. Hor. *Serm.* 2.16.19; Phaedr. 4.21.25–6; Suet. *Nero* 39.1). Valerius Maximus relates the generosity of the Roman undertakers in the matter of the funerals of Hirtius and Pansa in order to illustrate the idea that a place is reserved in the highest glory for even the most sordid favours and in rounding out the anecdote remarks that the humble condition of the protagonists increased rather than diminished their honour, inasmuch as 'those who live for nothing but profit [had] scorned profit' (5.2.10). There was nothing inherently ignoble in the activity of burying the dead – on the contrary, laying the dead to rest was a *negotium humanitatis* (*Dig.* 11.7.14.7 [Ulpian]). Ignominy lay in performing for pay what was regarded as a natural obligation of humanity.[8] Unlike the sordid occupations of prostitution, acting and serving as a gladiator, which permanently defiled those who practised them, and which for members of the higher orders brought down *infamia* and a diminution of status (cf. *Tab. Heracl.* 122–3; Edwards 1997), performing the duties of an undertaker disqualified a man from municipal office at Heraclea only so long as he was actively engaged in the practice.

On the other hand, the nature of the work, the business of caring for the dead, was regarded as inherently dirty, and death itself was religiously unclean. According to Plutarch (*Numa* 12.1), Numa taught the pontiffs not to regard burial rites as causing pollution, but any observer of the mortuary rituals surrounding a Roman funeral might be forgiven for concluding otherwise (see De Marchi 1896: 190–9; Scheid 1984: 118–20; Lindsay, in this volume). When a person died his family and household became *funesta* or *funestata* (Cic. *Leg.* 2.55; *Dig.* 45.3.28.4 [Gaius]; Gell. 4.6.8; Serv. ad *Aen.* 6.216, 3.64) a concept that is set in direct contrast by our literary sources with that of the *familia pura* (Varr. ap. Non. Marc. 240.18 L.). Until the completion of the cleansing rites, generally on the ninth day after the deposition of the body, various signs were posted to warn away those who wanted or who needed to remain pure: a cypress branch was planted outside the house door (Serv. ad *Aen.* 3.64; 6.216; cf. Hor. *Ep.* 5.18; Stat. *Theb.* 4.460–1.; Pliny *NH* 16.40, 139); flutes and horns playing a distinctive strain accompanied the corpse wherever it went (Festus p. 82 L.; Prop. 4.11.9–11); family members covered their hair with ashes (Catull. 64.351; Virg. *Aen.* 10.844, 12.611) and donned a specially darkened mourning gown, known variously as the *toga pulla* or *atra* (Paul. exc. Fest. p. 273 L.; Hor. *Ep.* 1.7.5; Tac. *Ann.* 3.2; Juv. 3.212; Cass. Dio 5.17.2) or, significantly *toga sordida* (*Dig.* 47.10.39 [Venuleius]; see further Heskell 1994: 141–2 on Cic. *Vat.* 30–2; *Sest.* 26, 32–3, 144–5); those who attended the funeral refrained from bathing (Petr. 42.1; Cic. *Vat.* 31; cf. Diod. Sic. 1.91.1); and upon their return underwent the cleansing rite known as *suffitio*, whereby they sprinkled themselves with water and walked over fire (Paul. exc. Fest. p. 3 L. s.v. 'Aqua et igni'); and so on (see Deschamps 1995: 172–4). It is not entirely clear for whom, among the general population, these warnings were intended, but magistrates and certain high priests, the Pontifex Maximus (Sen. *Cons. ad Marc.* 15.3) and Flamen Dialis in particular (Vanggaard 1988: 97; Lindsay, in this volume), were objects of special concern, since the religious purity of their persons was intimately bound up with the welfare of the state. It was to avoid inadvertently crossing their paths, according to one tradition, that Roman funerals were originally held at night ([Serv.] ad *Aen.* 11.143).

It is therefore not surprising to find epithets describing squalor and uncleanliness attaching to workers in the funerary trade: the corpse-burner is *sordidus* (Lucan 8.737; cf. Catul. 59.4); the name of the mortician, *pollinctor*, is said to derive from his role as a 'perfumer of the polluted', *pollutorum unctor* (Apul. *in Hermagor.*; ap. Fulg. *De serm. antiq.* 2; cf. Sidon. *Epist.* 3.13.5); even the funeral director, in Tertullian's jaundiced eyes (*Spect.* 10), is 'most foul', *inquinatissimus*. It follows too that funerary workers were for this reason among the most despised of wage-labourers: in astrological literature of the early Empire, they are classed with criminals in prison and prostitutes tied to the brothel as persons inseparably bound by their occupation to an unenviable and unclean mode of life (Firm. *Math.* 208, 20; Manetho 6.531–5; cf. Cumont 1937: 142 n. 2). Unclean, it should be noted, in a physical and possibly a moral sense, but not for that reason polluted in religious terms. The fourth-century astrologer Manetho says explicitly that funerary workers in Egypt were shunned because they were *asemnoi*, which in his day did not so much mean 'unholy' as 'indecent' or 'obscene' (*Apotelesmata* 4.190; cf. *LSJ* s.v.). Already by the end of the second century BC a local decree at Thebes had ordered the embalmers to quit the community and to take up residence in the necropolis across the river (*UPZ* II.162 col. 4.28–9 with Wilcken's remarks *ad loc.* and on p. 39). The mandate originated with the town doctor and is perhaps therefore more likely to have been motivated by considerations of health, or possibly amenity, than by religious concerns: the stench produced by the embalmers' work was notoriously offensive (see Perdrizet 1934: 724–6). It is worth noting, moreover, that at around this same time the embalmers of Oxyrhynchus were living as and among ordinary members of the community (*P. Tebt.* III.967; cf. Derda 1991: 20 and n. 41). These sorts of regulations, in other words, were local and might vary from place to place. Whereas Martial encountered tattooed corpse-bearers in the streets of

Rome (Mart. 8.75.9), at Puteoli the contracting undertaker was forbidden to employ workmen with tattoos (*AE* 1971, 88 II.7) – presumably in order to exclude criminals and slaves of proven bad character (Jones 1987). This should warn us against assuming too great a uniformity in the details of local regulations governing the conduct of workers in the funerary trade.

Certain broad trends can nevertheless be discerned. One of these, across the empire, was toward an increasing segregation of corpse-handlers from the rest of society in isolated communities on the outskirts of town. At Puteoli, funerary workers were prohibited from entering the town except on official business and were forbidden to live closer to town than a tower where the local Grove of Libitina was located (*AE* 1971, 88 II.3–4).[9] We have already mentioned the removal of local embalmers at Egyptian Thebes from the town centre to the necropolis across the river, and astrological literature of the early Empire shows that cemetery guards regularly dwelled among the tombs they were hired to protect, outside the community of the living (Cumont 1937: 141 n. 1). In Egypt the term *exōpulitēs*, 'a dweller outside the gates', attested in a dozen ostraka and papyri dating from the third to the eighth century, came to be used generically of any of the various workers in the funerary trade, who were so-called because they lived apart, in segregated communities outside the towns they served (Youtie 1973). And at Constantinople, the emperor Constantine established a formal corporation of *lecticarii*, headquartered in the suburbs, whose job it was to oversee burials and to transport the corpses of the indigent, free of charge, to the grave (Justinian *Nov.* 43 praef., 59 praef.; cf. Rush 1941: 204).

It is difficult to know whether certain other restrictions imposed on funerary workers at Puteoli were generally applicable or were locally specific. At times the motives underlying them seem to have been contradictory. A clause requiring the undertaker's staff to wear distinctive clothing (a dark-coloured cap, *pilleus coloratus*), for example, and to refrain from bathing after the first hour of the night, likens funerary workers to those in mourning (*AE* 1971, 88 II.4–6). In a sense, their daily contact with death seems to have consigned them to a permanent state of sordidness. A clause from the same paragraph requiring the undertaker's workmen to be free of disfiguring marks and physical imperfections, on the other hand, points to a very different condition (*AE* 1971, 88 II.6–7). As is well known, sacrificial animals were regarded as unsuitable for offering to the gods unless free from blemishes, and certain Roman priests, notably Vestal Virgins, for whom the requirements of purity were especially stringent, had likewise to be physically intact in order to assume their priesthoods (cf. Dion. Hal. *Ant. Rom.* 2.21.3; Sen. *Contr.* 4.2; Gell. 1.12.3; Fronto, p. 142 Van den Hout with Gwyn Morgan 1974). Plutarch remarks upon the obvious similarity between the two requirements and speculates that Roman practice forbade bodily imperfections in persons or things involved in sacred matters (*Quaest Rom.* 73 = *Mor.* 281C; cf. Leviticus 21.16–24). Strictly, in Roman sacral law the business of burying the dead fell under the heading of *res religiosae* rather than *res sacrae*, but the evidence from Puteoli suggests that in the matter of physical purity the two spheres overlapped. Whatever the precise implications of this shared concern, nothing could better illustrate the ambivalence of Roman attitudes toward those responsible for caring for the dead than the combination of this requirement of physical integrity, which likens workers in the funerary trade to the sort of priests for whom purity was at a premium, and the popular revulsion from their persons, which were regarded as more or less permanently soiled through habitual contact with the dead (cf. Hinard 1995: 211).

Executioners

Defer, defer
to the Lord High Executioner
W. S. Gilbert, *The Mikado*

No such ambiguity surrounds the figure of the executioner: the Roman verdict on his status was unequivocal and unanimous. As a purveyor of death, he was both physically abhorrent and religiously dangerous. The latter quality in particular derived from the nature of his work. Whereas all those who handled dead bodies were made unclean by direct contact with decomposing human flesh, executioners bore the additional burden of serving as the instruments of a rite of excommunication from the community. According to an old and well-established principle of Roman penal law, persons condemned to death for violations against the state, and hence for threatening the *pax deorum*, were devoted to some god or other, usually to the gods of the underworld, so that the Roman people should not suffer divine punishment. The offender became a *homo sacer* and could be killed with impunity (Dion. Hal. *Ant. Rom.* 2.10.3; Livy 3.55.5; cf. Mommsen 1899: 900–4). Festus notes the paradox that it was not right that the offender be sacrificed to the gods, although, as an outlaw, he could justifiably be killed (Fest. p. 424 L.), and Macrobius explains why this was so: the only way a god could claim retribution from an offender was by taking his soul; thus the execution of a condemned man was simply a means of severing the soul from the body in order to deliver it to the injured party for punishment (Macrob. 3.7.5–7; cf. [Serv.] ad *Aen.* 10.419; Cantarella 1991: 303–5). The name *carnifex*, literally 'meat-maker' (Donat. ad *Ter. Hec.* 441; Isid. *Etym.* 10.49), reflects this conception of the executioner's role as that of one who separates spirit from flesh, rendering of a human mere meat (for *caro* in opposition to *anima*, cf. *OLD* s.v. 2b).

As the agent of delivery, the executioner came into contact with a person formally exiled from the community; consequently, according to Roman notions of contagion, he was inevitably infected with the pollution of his victim and therefore, like the victim, had to be shunned. Cicero makes this concept of contagion abundantly clear when he writes, in his defence of C. Rabirius, that he refuses to allow the assembly of the Roman people to be polluted (*funestari*) by contact with the executioner and declares that the Forum must be purified (*expiandum*) of his presence (*Rab. perd.* 11). The same idea underlies the premise of a declamation reported by Calpurnius Flaccus in which a son condemned to death by a father exercising *patria potestas* accepts the sentence but objects to the insult of dying at the hands of the public executioner: let the father slay the victim he has vowed to the household gods, so long as he does not contaminate the law of piety by consigning the act to the vile hand of a contemptible man (*Decl.* 24 with Sussman 1994: 168 *ad loc.*; cf. Curt. *Alex.* 8.2.2, *detestabile carnificis ministerium*). That this abhorrence of the executioner derived from a perception of his impurity is indicated by an analogy preserved in another declamation of Calpurnius' and drawn from the same realm of sacrifice: 'no one takes a victim from a polluted herd (*de polluto grege*): who will dispatch such a victim? a father? a priest? or an executioner (*carnifex*)?' (*Decl.* 44).

Recognising this perception of the executioner as a carrier of pollution helps to explain why Roman authors so frequently express their revulsion explicitly in terms of avoiding physical contact with his person, and especially with his hands, the most active vehicles of contamination.[10] It also explains why executioners were barred from living in the community. According to Cicero, the regulations of the censors forbade the executioner not only to reside in the city and to frequent the Forum but to look upon the same sky and to breathe the same air as other urban residents (Cic. *Rab. perd.* 15; cf. § 10). Here we must allow for rhetorical exaggeration. Plautus tells us exactly where the public torturers and executioners were to be found: outside the town gates (Plaut. *Pseud.* 331–2; cf. *Mil.* 359; Sen. *Contr.* 1.2.21). Just outside, he implies, whence they could be summoned on short notice. At Rome, it seems a reasonable inference that the Esquiline Gate is meant (Wiseman 1985: 7–8). A place was set aside on the Esquiline for servile punishments – crucifixion, burning alive and precipitation from a height – and it was there, it seems, in the vicinity of the *puticuli*, at a place known as *Sessorium*, that the corpses of those denied formal burial rites were abandoned to the dogs and birds.[11] Nearby were sandpits where in the time of Sulla a young man from Larinum was murdered (Cic. *Clu.* 37). No wonder the Romans dedicated an altar of Misfortune in the vicinity (Pliny *NH* 2.16). When Martial and Juvenal mention executioners together with corpse-bearers (*vespillones*) and coffin-makers (*fabri sandapilarum*), they may therefore have been acknowledging a topographical as well as a conceptual connection among them (Mart. 2.61.3–4; Juv. 8.175–6). A confused scholion on Horace's satire about Maecenas' suburban *horti* represents executioners actually digging *puticuli* in the Esquiline road ([Acro] ad Hor. *Sat.* 1.8.10). This curious conflation perhaps finds some support in the mortuary arrangements at Puteoli, where the contracting undertaker was obliged to maintain floggers and an executioner on his staff, who were subject to the same living conditions as the other workmen (*AE* 1971, 88 II.8–14).

But if the Puteolan law illustrates a close and natural association of funerary tradesmen and executioners, it also highlights a fundamental difference between them. It was suggested above that the clause prohibiting funerary workers from bathing after the first hour of the night and requiring them to wear dark caps when in town likens them to persons in mourning: manifest signs of uncleanliness set them apart from society at large and from the corpse in particular, which, washed and perfumed and dressed in white, was being separated from the world of the living through a series of purificatory rites (Rush 1941: 126–7; Scheid 1984: 120–1). The executioner, by contrast, through his contact with a person already divorced from the community of the living by the imposition of a death sentence, is forced to share in the condemned's outlaw status. Thus he is made to resemble his victim. This seems to be what Festus alludes to when he writes that those who wound themselves mortally are considered to have taken on the role of executioner: the act of a bloody suicide mirrors the assimilation of the *carnifex* to the condemned in that both executioner and victim are sullied by the killing.[12]

At Puteoli a workman ordered to haul away the corpse of an executed criminal with a hook 'to where there will be more corpses' was required to dress in red (*russatus*) and to ring a bell while performing the task (*AE* 1971, 88 II.13–14). Both details point to this assimilation. Romans of the classical period would probably have associated garments of the dark brownish hue described by the adjectives *russus* and *russeus* with the colour of blood-stains produced in combat. A scholion on the *Aeneid* tells us that Roman soldiers used to dress in red before entering battle in order to conceal the evidence of wounds and the inevitable bespatterings of blood, whence they came to be called *russati*, 'the reddened ones', or 'the ones dressed in red'.[13] Whatever the reliability of this testimony, which found its way also into the etymological encyclopedia of Isidore of Seville (*Orig.* 19.22.10), Tertullian speaks of a soldier being reddened, *russatus*, with his own blood (*Coron. Mil.* 1.3), and we may compare the practice of Roman *triumphatores* of smearing their faces with earth of Sinope or cinnabar 'instead of blood' (*anti haimatos*) in order to screen their blushes (Tzetzes *Epist.* 107, p. 86; cf. *Chil.* 13, 43–4). It seems reasonable to conclude that the Puteolan corpse-dragger's russet clothing was in some sense perceived to be emblematic of his occupation of butchery. His uniform reflected the condition of his victim: both were the colour of blood.

The corpse-dragger's bell points to a similar connection. A pair of passages of Plautus shows that the association of executioners with bells was both old and well-established in Roman culture. In *Pseudolus*, the slave protagonist responds to his master's injunction to prepare for a sacrifice by promising to fetch two 'butchers with bells' (*lanii … cum tintinnabulis*) from beyond the gate to extract the sacrificial blood with birch rods; the context makes it clear that he is referring to the local floggers (*Pseud.* 331–2). Elsewhere Plautus coins a term *tintinnaculi*, 'the ringers', to refer obliquely to the public executioners and expects his audience to make the identification: so strong was the popular association of bells and torturers in his day that no glossing of the new term was required (*Truc.* 781–2). A passage of Cassius Dio epitomised by Zonaras illuminates the origin of the connection: in explaining why a bell and whip were fastened to the Roman triumphal chariot, Zonaras says that it was customary for those who had been condemned to die to wear a bell, 'so that no one should approach them as they walked along and become contaminated with pollution' (Zon. *Epit.* 7.21). No doubt the bells carried by Plautus' executioners and the Puteolan corpse-hauler were likewise intended to serve as a defensive precaution against accidental pollution. All those involved in the physical separation of a condemned outlaw from the community of the living were tainted, and persons who needed or wanted to remain pure were warned away at their approach.

Whether the bells fulfilled their original purpose in Plautus' time and later, however, is another question. Just as the blare of an ambulance siren nowadays awakens in some a morbid curiosity to rush to the scene of the car wreck, so the executioner's bell is as likely to have attracted spectators as to have turned them away. Literary testimony makes it clear that the sight of a mangled corpse dragged off by the hook was a popular spectacle, eliciting applause from the crowd (e.g. Cic. *Verr.* 5.65; Juv. 10.66; Cass. Dio 58.11.5 [Sejanus]; Ovid, *Ibis* 165; Cat. 108 with Wiseman 1985: 6–7). Public gloating over the corpse seems to have satisfied a popular thirst for vengeance (e.g. [Quint.] *Decl. Min.* 247.18, 274.7) and in some no doubt exacerbated a more primal blood-lust, or at any rate a morbid fascination. Herein lies the essential paradox of the executioner's role: although he carried pollution and was treated as a pariah, his public performances were eagerly viewed. Plato's anecdote about the reluctant corpse-watcher Leontius provides the classic illustration of this fundamental human conflict between illicit desire and moral revulsion: when returning one day from the Piraeus Leontius encountered an executioner standing over the bodies of some criminals lying on the ground; unable to resist the urge to stare but disgusted by the prospect, he finally rushed over to feast his eyes, cursing them all the while (*Rep.* 4.439e–440a).

In a Roman context the ambivalence exhibited toward the executioner manifested itself in popular attitudes toward gladiators as well, some of whom were called upon to dispatch condemned criminals at the midday shows. As genuine combatants who put their lives at risk, gladiators enjoyed a glamour and romantic appeal of which the public executioner had no part (Hopkins 1983: 20–7; Barton 1993: 11–46); at the same time, their occupation of homicide implicated them in the same pollution as the executioner and reinforced their seclusion from the rest of society (cf. Aigner 1988: 201–9). A well-known inscription of late Republican date from Sarsina in Umbria explicitly excludes paid gladiators, suicides by hanging, and 'those who have practiced a sordid profession' from burial in a private plot donated to the community (*CIL* I^2 2123 = XI 6528 = *ILS* 7846 = *ILLRP* 662; cf. Susini 1969; Hope, in this volume). More pointedly, at Rhodes, according to Dio of Prusa, the Rhodians banished gladiators from their community on the grounds that their laws also forbade executioners from entering the city (Dio Chrys. *Or.* 31.123; cf. Ville 1981: 340–1, 462–3). At Rome the residential restrictions imposed on gladiators seem not to have been so severe, but their barracks, at least from the time of Domitian, were constructed in such a way that their inhabitants could move back and forth from their quarters to their place of work, the Flavian amphitheatre, without coming into contact with the general population (Colini and Cozza 1962). This precaution may have been motivated primarily by concerns for the physical safety of the populace, but it served as well to protect the surrounding community from the pollution carried by those engaged in the business of killing.

Conclusion

Three views of the Roman conception of death-pollution, which have focused on the provisions made for the burial of the poor at Rome and on the attitudes and behaviour displayed toward the professionals responsible for conducting funerals and performing public executions, illustrate a range of responses. When it came to disposing of the dead in public facilities, the Romans were content to put aside their religious precepts regarding the sanctity of graves and approached the problem exclusively in terms of pragmatic considerations of hygiene and amenity. In their treatment of undertakers and other workers in the funerary trade, a natural aversion to the physically dirty aspects of their work seems to shade into a more ambivalent recognition of their function as mediators between the worlds of the living and the dead, a role which links them with those in mourning as fellow participants in the series of purificatory rituals designed to effect the transition from one state to the other. Executioners, as purveyors of death and agents of the formal severing of an outcast from the community, are not only morally abhorrent but religiously impure and thus potentially dangerous vehicles of pollution; and yet, the Roman passion for blood spectacle cast them also in the role of popular entertainers.

What this preliminary investigation suggests, then, is that our approach to understanding Roman ways of dealing with the dead needs to be more alert to ambiguity and ambivalence than it traditionally has been; it should take account of practical as well as spiritual and 'religious' considerations as determinants of Roman behaviour; it should recognise the various modes of assimilation and integration of professional and private participants in the mortuary ritual; and it should weigh carefully the competing impulses of revulsion and fascination in its assessment of the popular response to the spectacle of public executions. The view offered here from the bottom up thus presents a more variegated, less sharply defined picture of Roman attitudes than that afforded by our upper-class literary authorities. If it appears less clear and bright than the uplifting images painted by a Polybius or a Cicero, it may nevertheless claim to reflect more truly the grey realities of Roman life, where the graves of the poor were not graves at all, where undertakers and morticians were shunned as unclean, yet played indispensable roles in the purifying rituals that separated the living from the dead, and where executioners resembling their victims were simultaneously objects of loathing and purveyors of entertainment.

Acknowledgements

An earlier version of this chapter benefited from the comments of attentive participants at the conference on 'Pollution and the Ancient City' at Exeter University and at a meeting of the New England Ancient History Colloquium at Amherst College. I am especially grateful for helpful suggestions to Carlin Barton, Kathleen Coleman, W. T. Loomis and Stephen Todd, and to David Noy for sharing with me his forthcoming essay on Roman cremations gone awry.

NOTES

1 Attempting to identify this most wretched segment of the urban plebs on the basis of the pejorative epithets sometimes applied to it by ancient writers (e.g. *plebs sordida*, *infima plebs*, *inops vulgus*) is fruitless: see Yavetz 1969: 141–55. Criminals, suicides by hanging, those who practised dishonourable professions, and any who had enemies in power, might fear even worse post-mortem fates: mutilation of their corpses and denial of burial: see Hope, in this volume.

2 If N = 750,000 (= *c.* 4.25 × 175,000, a crude average of the estimated population figures at the beginning and end of the nineteenth century), then, without accounting for a higher mortality rate in the denser and larger urban population of ancient Rome, we arrive at *c.* 17,000–25,500 deaths annually ([4,000–6,000] × 4.25), rising to 51,000 (12,000 × 4.25) in times of plague. The bibliography on urban mortality is vast: two volumes of *Annales de démographie historique* (1962, 1978) provide a conspectus of views on the issue as of twenty years ago, and interest in the topic has grown since then: see, e.g., Wrigley 1987: 147 n. 12.

3 When coffins were used, naturally the capacity of these mass graves was reduced. At one churchyard in central London in 1774 the poor were buried in pits 'capable of holding three or four coffins abreast and about seven in depth' (Gittings 1984: 64). Prior to the sanitary regulations of the 1840s, common graves in England were often filled with three coffins abreast, stacked twelve deep (Laqueur 1983: 116). At Hart Island in New York, where the coffins are set in place by a back hoe, the burial trenches measure forty by fifteen feet in area and ten feet in depth (Conlan 1993: 51). Lanciani's estimate (1890: 65–6) that a section of the trench outside the Servian *agger* just north of the Esquiline Gate (cf. Bodel 1994: 109–10 n. 165) measuring approximately 160 × 100 × 30 feet

(i.e. 480,000 cubic feet) and filled to the top with corpses contained some 24,000 bodies assumes an improbably large number of cubic feet (20) per corpse. If the density of burials was similar to that found in the mass-grave pits of early modern Europe (*c.* 7.5–8 cubic feet per corpse), the trench would have held some 60,000 to 64,000 bodies.

4 It is tempting to associate the construction, at precisely the second mile of the Via Prenestina, of the huge, late Republican or early Augustan tumulus tomb (42 metres in diameter) known as the 'Torrione' with this decree of the senate: see Pietrangeli 1940. To the best of my knowledge, mass burial pits on the outskirts of Rome are not found again before the Christian era after Constantine, when, for example, a series of pits capable of containing fifty or more corpses was installed in the cemetery of Commodilla: Josi 1950: 1626. These *pozzi* are in any case on a different scale from the vast *puticuli* of the Republican period.

5 For practices outside Roman towns, see Bodel 1994: 81–3. To the arguments there adduced in favour of Pascal's etymology of *cula* at Agenn. Urb. *Corp. Agr.* p. 47 Th. (below n. 11) from the Greek, *koila*, 'underground cavities', add the testimony of Strabo 8.5.7, discussing the execution pit outside Sparta known as the Kaiadas: 'some prefer to call such cavernous hollows (*koilōmata*) "kōoi", whence the expression "oreskōioi", "monsters" (see Hom. *Il.* 1.268). From *kōoi* and *koilōmata* to *koila* is an easy route, and the appropriateness of the term in context in Agennius (*habent et loca noxiorum poenis destinata*) is apparent.

6 See further Thompson 1988: 155–7, on the difficulty of discerning the precise functions behind the Greek terms by which Egyptian funerary workers are generally known to us, and Montserrat 1997, on the two stages of Egyptian funerals, the *peristolē* and the *kēdeia*, describing, respectively, the periods before and after the processing of the corpse.

7 *CIL* I^2 593.94–6 *neve quis que<i> praeconium dissignationem libitinamve faciet, dum eorum quid faciet, in muni/cipio colonia praefectura IIvir(atum) IIIIvir(atum) aliumve quem mag(istratum) petito neve capito neve gerito neve habeto,/neve ibei senator neve decurio neve conscriptus esto neve sententiam dicito.*

8 In contemporary Cantonese society, the full purification of death-pollution requires that someone accept money for performing part of the funerary ritual. Specifically, paid surrogates are required to take on voluntarily the baleful effects of 'killing airs': cf. Watson 1988: 111, 114–15. Livy 7.2.12 implies that attitudes toward actors and acting were governed by a similar distinction: what mattered was whether or not the performers were paid: see Gardner 1993: 140.

9 *AE* 1971, 88 II.3–4, *Oper(ae) quae at eam r(em) praeparat(ae) er(unt) ne intra turrem ubi hodie lucus est Libit(inae) habitent laventurve ab h(ora) I noctis, neve veniant in oppid(um) nisi mortui tollend(i) conlocand(i)ve aut supplic(i) sumend(i) c(ausa).* For the sense of the phrase *intra turrem* adopted here, see Bodel 1994: 95–6 n. 61. Dumont 1995: 181–2 believes that the workmen were prohibited from living inside a tower of the town wall, Hinard 1995: 208–10 that they were excluded from a grove in an elevated location outside the town.

10 Cf., e.g., Cic. *2 Ver.* 5.113 [cf. Sen. *Contr.* 2.5.2]; Sen. *Contr.* 1.3.1, 2.3.19, 9.2.3 [cf. Exc. 9.2.1–2]; Ovid, *Ibis* 165; Val. Max. 6.9.13, 7.2 (Ext.).1, 9.12.6; Sil. *Pun.* 1.172; Pliny *Ep.* 4.11.9; Tac. *Ann.* 6.39.2; Calp. Flacc. *Decl.* 24; Apul. *Met.* 9.1.1; [Quint.] *Decl. Min.* 277.2 (cf. 277.3), 372.7; *Decl. Mai.* 11.10. Catullus 97.11–12 invokes an even less clean part of the executioner's anatomy.

11 Tac. *Ann.* 15.60.2; Sessorium: [Acro] Hor. *Epode* 5.100; if the text of Plut. *Galbaad* 28.2–3 is emended correctly, those put to death by the emperors were abandoned there. See further Hinard 1987: 113–15. The establishment outside Roman towns, near the public facilities for burying the indigent, of specific areas for the punishment of criminals, seems to have been normal: Agenn. Urb. *De controv. agror.* (*Corp. Agr.* p. 47 Th.): *habent et res p(ublicae) loca suburbana inopum funeribus destinata, quae loca †cula culinas† appellant. Habent et loca noxiorum poenis destinata* (see above, n. 5).

12 Paul exc. Fest. p. 56 L. The assimilation of the executioner to his victim is well noted by David 1984: 144, who interprets Festus' remark to mean that the executioner's corpse, like that of a suicide, is denied burial (so also Aigner 1988: 202–3). Professor Kathleen Coleman suggests (*per litteras*) that someone who commits suicide is like an executioner in that he performs a rationally sanctioned act of killing. But among suicides, only those who hanged themselves were regularly denied burial (see Desideri 1995; Kyle 1998: 131–2, with further references), and the point of Festus' remark seems to hinge on the verb *vulnerare*, which implies bloodshed.

13 *Trosula quae purpura cocoque pretexta conficitur cui idcirco coccum adhibetur quod russati antea proeliabantur propter vulnera et aspersiones sanguinis, quo posset hoc colore velari, unde russati vocabantur.* Preserved in this form in the margin of the Tours manuscript of Servius Danielis (Bern. 165) at *Aen.* 7.612, the scholion seems to have been known also to Scaliger, who may have acquired its exemplar from Daniel (so Thilo 173).

11

DEATH-POLLUTION AND FUNERALS IN THE CITY OF ROME

Hugh Lindsay

Introduction

The aim of this chapter is to examine some of the complex factors shaping Roman funerary practices. Aspects of Roman customs show fear or at least avoidance of close contact with death. From the time of the Twelve Tables, and perhaps earlier, the place of burial had been regulated, distancing the living and the dead. Moreover, while intimate family had an inevitable involvement in the death of a relative, for outsiders death involved some ambiguity, especially in their dealings with the bereaved family. A distance, both spatial and temporal, could be observed between the corpse and the family on the one hand and the outside world on the other. Why was this the case? Reasons for shunning family members may often be complex; these could include feelings of respect for the deceased, or sensitivity to the family's need for space to cope with the death. Other reasons may have been motivated by fear or insecurities; to see the dead and the bereaved was to be reminded of one's own mortality. In addition the corpse, and those in close proximity to it, may have been viewed as in some way polluted or contaminated by death. It is this concept of death-pollution, and how it was manifested in the Roman context, which lies at the heart of this chapter.

Roman ideas about the concept of death-pollution may be important to understanding Roman institutions. Modern approaches to the whole area of pollution have noted that there is an overlap between religious and non-religious ideas of contagion, and this approach is also relevant to the pollution deriving from a death (Douglas 1968: 336–40). Death-pollution can be identified as follows. A fear of death-pollution is a product of the bad omen represented by a death. In societies where belief in death-pollution is strong, it is held that the corpse has the power to contaminate those who, in various ways, come close. It can be a spiritual pollution related to the need for the soul of the deceased to be placated through appropriate funerary rites, but it may have a physical dimension. Physical proximity, secondary contact (e.g. sighting a corpse), and, most dangerously, touching the corpse can result in contamination (Watson 1988: 112–13). This concern with contamination is thus related to both the material world and religious belief. Mary Douglas has shown that a rigid distinction between religious and secular behaviour in relation to pollution may be misleading. The behavioural reactions to pollution can be seen as attempts to reduce dissonance in the aftermath of an event which 'is likely to confuse or contradict cherished classifications' (Douglas 1968: 340). Thus in our interpretation of Roman customs, concerns over pollution need not centre on spiritual thinking, but can also relate to more practical concern over the disintegration of the body of the deceased.

It will be argued here that the Roman habit of keeping death at arm's length from the city was not exclusively dominated by either religious or hygienic considerations; rather both practical concerns about the health of the urban environment and the remnants of age-old taboos mutually reinforced one another. Although some signs of concern over spiritual pollution can be detected in Roman society, it would be a misguided approach to overplay this element, when we consider the diversity of belief about the fate of the human soul in the world of the late Republic and early Empire.

In the following discussion I shall investigate three main themes. The first will be the social impact of death-pollution. Here the aim will be to look at the standing of the family in which a death has occurred and the impact the death has on the family's dealings with the wider community. The interesting taboos relating to magistrates and funeral professionals are at the core of this section. In the second section the rituals of transition will be scrutinised. A chronological account of the main features reported by literary sources will proceed from the deathbed scene to the grave. This section is partly descriptive, but also aims to identify elements in the rituals which seem to have evolved from a concern with death-pollution. The methods employed by the family to purge the pollution after the funeral are also examined, as well as the relative merits of inhumation and incineration. The final part of the chapter has a limited scope. It will discuss the little that is known about legislation relating to the location of graves. Here the purpose will be to try to identify the issues addressed by the legislators, and specifically whether they were more concerned over hygiene or spiritual pollution. Clearly this will leave open the important question of where the Romans actually disposed of their dead. This has been discussed by other contributors in this volume (Patterson; Hope).

In all three sections literary, epigraphic and archaeological evidence has been employed, and this has its own hazards; the combination of different types of evidence may result in gross simplifications, or loss of original context and purpose. Moreover, it is difficult to produce an image of Roman funerary practices which is clearly applicable to a single time and place. The combination of diverse material risks creating an amalgamated picture, parts of which may in fact have evolved over time. There is the further danger that aristocratic habits will be over-represented; in general the quality of our coverage allows for little differentiation of status, and funerals in poorer families do not emerge in detail. My aim has been to centre on the period 200 BC to AD 200, and to place the primary focus on the city of Rome.[1] Despite all the chronological and spatial difficulties alluded to above it seems valid to identify some continuities in funerary practices which are illustrative of concerns over death-pollution.

The social impact of death-pollution

A death in the family and the advent of pollution

Pollution would fall upon the house and family of a deceased Roman from the time of death. The household would be subject to mourning (*funesta*) and, according to the fourth-century Servius, a person in mourning (*funestatus*) was not entitled to sacrifice to the gods (Servius *ad Aen.* 11.2). Varro, writing in the age of Caesar, believed this period of mourning was brought to a conclusion by the inhumation of the body (Varro *Ling.* 5.23), but this may be misleading. As will be seen below, the final purificatory act in the rite of passage of the deceased is the sacrifice on the ninth day after death (*novemdial sacrificium*). Servius in a number of passages insists that in earlier times Romans had strong reactions to a death in the family, and identifies certain precautions that were taken to avert the consequences of pollution. Some ambiguity must remain over whether pollution is the main or sole issue; since mourning also involves issues of respect for the deceased and those who are close to him.

Servius describes how pontifical law stepped in to avert some of the more extreme consequences that could have flowed from the pollution which fell on a household where a death had taken place (Serv. *ad Aen.* 6.8). For example, in ignorance of the death in the family, a family member who was a *pontifex* could have offered a sacrifice to the gods before the household had been purified. In such a case pontifical law would decree that the *funestatio* (mourning for a death) did not begin until the death was acknowledged by the head of the family (*funus agnoscere*). If the *pontifex* heard news of a death during a sacrifice, in other words after the ritual acts had begun, he had to retain this information until the sacrifice was completed (Serv. *ad Aen.* 11.2; Livy 2.8.7). This subsequently became a precedent for the idea that a religious act once begun could not be invalidated by the arrival of news of ill omen during its performance (Cic. *Domo* 138–9). It is also of interest to note that the death of a child who had not reached puberty was considered not to entail a pollution in the house provided that the body was carried off at night. Servius says that when the children of magistrates died, they were removed with particular care (Serv. *ad Aen.* 11.143). The attitude to infants appears to be closely related both to ideas about when a child is integrated into the household (*familia*) and thus seen as a full member of the community, and to Roman ideas about the development of the soul (see Flower 1996: 97).

To indicate a house of death during the period of exposition of the body branches of pine (*picea*) or cypress were planted in front of the door of the house. The cypress was used because once cut it would not regrow, and was thus considered sacred to Dis, the god of the underworld, and the Roman equivalent of Pluto (Plin. *NH* 16.40; 16.139; Festus-Paulus 56L s.v. 'cupressus'; Hor. *Od.* 2.14.23). According to Servius, the marking of the death-house was intended as a warning of possible pollution which had special relevance for the pontiffs. Any form of contact with or sight of a corpse was thought to entail pollution and Servius claims that the Romans took particular care to keep these priests away from the sources of trouble, so that they could continue to exercise their duties in relation to public cults (Serv. *ad Aen.* 3.64). Pliny, in referring to these pine and cypress branches, does not mention this pollution angle, and Servius may be providing antiquarian material.

Servius thought that funerals in the earliest days of the city took place at night under torchlight to protect priests such as the pontiffs and the priest of Jupiter (*flamen Dialis*) from the danger of pollution (Serv. *ad Aen.* 1.727, 6.224, 11.143; Rushton 1915: 149–64). Some confusion based on these passages in Servius has crept into modern authorities, but it seems unlikely that the original funeral ceremony was ever held at night (Rose 1923: 191–4).

Torches made of ropes or firebands (*funes* or *faces*) always remained customary for the *funus acerbum* (a painful funeral) – that of a child. This was held at night but it was a special case that did not involve disposal of an acknowledged social personality (Cuq 1881: s.v. 'funus' 1390; Boyancé 1952: 275–89; Néraudau 1984: 375ff.). A consequence was that very young children could be buried within the city limits. There is evidence of the burial of children in the Forum and on the Palatine dating from as early as the seventh century BC (Néraudau ibid.; Schilling 1976: 947ff.). In the case of children's funerals in the age of Seneca candles were used for lighting (Sen. *Ep.* 122; *Tranq.* 11; *De Brev. Vitae* 20; *Hercules Furens* 849ff.). By this stage it is clear that children were normally buried along with adults. The most likely explanation of the illumination is apotropaic, but it also has importance in enabling the living to stay away from the pollution that they would undergo were they to see the corpse. Night funerals might also be thought of as preventing something impure from appearing in the light of day (De Visscher 1963: 35–6). But, in general, adult funerals were conducted during daylight hours (Hor. *Serm.* 1.6.42; Plut. *Sulla* 38; *CIL* VI 13782). The tradition of carrying torches to light the convoy was thus not directly related to illumination, any more than on the occasion of marriages or births.

Further measures were employed to keep the priestly class away from death-pollution. There was a taboo on eating, touching or even naming beans which applied to the priest of Jupiter (*flamen Dialis*) (Pötscher 1968: 215–39; Holleman 1973: 222–8; Boels 1973: 77–100). Pliny explains that beans are the souls (*animae*) of the dead, and for this reason are consumed on the *Parentalia*, an annual festival reserved for private celebrations of rites for the family dead (13–21 February). Messages from the dead (*lugubres litterae*) were also thought to appear on the flowers of bean runners (Pliny *NH* 18.118–19; Festus-Paulus 77L). Nevertheless, despite the taboo, it was not forbidden for the *flamen Dialis* to follow a funeral convoy (Fabius Pictor in Aulus Gellius *NA* 10.15; Cic. *Tusc.* 1.16).

Additional evidence on the danger of polluting priests through exposure to a corpse is provided by certain funerals associated with the imperial family. Dio comments that in 12 BC Augustus hung a curtain in front of the corpse of Agrippa before delivering his funeral speech (*laudatio*), but professes uncertainty over why he did this. He then discusses the possibility that it was a response to the danger of pollution in view of his status as *pontifex maximus* or *censor*, only to reject it. It would seem that Dio suffers from confusion because death-pollution was not much of an issue in his own day. He points out that a censor is only forbidden to view a corpse when he is about to complete the census, surely reflecting relaxations in practice current in the Severan era (Dio 54.28.4–5). We may wonder whether Augustus did not engage in this careful procedure as an advertisement of his acquisition of the status of *pontifex maximus* in 12 BC following the death of Lepidus (RG 10.2). The procedure could be deliberately archaising (cf. Price 1987: 66).

In the Julio-Claudian period we can note further examples where priests are expected to be excluded from contact with death. At the time of the death of Augustus, Tiberius was one of the pontiffs, and we learn from Dio that he was granted an indemnity for his contact with the corpse, and his involvement in the convoy to Rome (Dio 56.31.3). A key example of the behaviour expected from priests is the case of Germanicus in Germany, and his handling of the remains of the victims of the Varian disaster. He was at this time *augur*. In relation to this, Tacitus includes, as a motive for Tiberian disapproval of the interment of the relics, the fact that a general invested with the augurate ought not to have polluted himself by contact with funerary rites (Tac. *Ann.* 1.62; cf. Suet. *Calig.* 3). Tiberius appears to have been unusually particular about the dangers of death-pollution, since it attracts comment that when he was *pontifex maximus* he interposed a veil while pronouncing the funeral speech in commemoration of his son Drusus in order to prevent pollution from the sight of the corpse (Sen. *Cons. ad Marc.* 15.3). This can also be seen as an example of Tiberius' very careful pursuit of Augustan precedents. Clearly from a modern perspective there would always have been contradictions in Roman attitudes, since magistrates who commanded armies often held religious offices, but seem not to have been considered polluted as a result of the slaughter of the enemy. This may be related to the concept of a just war (*iustum bellum*), which effectively authorised the slaughter.

Funeral professionals at Rome

Some communities regard those involved in the undertaking trade as seriously tainted, that is permanently spiritually or physically polluted by contact with the dead. This approach seems to be strongest amongst ancestor worshippers, who see the power of the ancestor as closely connected to his links with the spirit world. Cantonese examples show that the period after death is seen as a liminal state during which the deceased is transformed from a dangerous corpse into a settled ancestor, and thus those who make their living from death are seen as existing in what amounts to a permanent state of liminality (Watson 1988: 130). As a result the Cantonese see funeral specialists as especially polluted. It is hard to prove that ancestor worship was ever conducted in Roman society, but some authorities have thought this probable (Lindsay 1996: 271–85; cf. Flower 1996). If ancestor worship was of importance in earlier phases of Roman development, residual elements from this phase might be expected to have endured. It may be of interest to compare the conduct of a funeral at Rome with that of an undoubted ancestor-worshipping society such as the Cantonese. I have argued recently that this is of special interest even though it is clear that far more extreme attitudes to pollution are manifested in the Chinese material (Lindsay 1998: 70). In Cantonese society there is the advantage that ancestor worship is not remote, and the purpose of each stage is easier to ascertain.

In Cantonese society a proper funeral can only take place if the bereaved are prepared to pay for the services of funeral specialists, specialists in 'white affairs', *pai shih*: white is the colour of mourning (Watson 1988: 109–34). The funeral professionals are ranked in proportion to their contact with the corpse. Those with the lowest ranking are the menials who handle the corpse and deal with materials closely associated with death. Distinctions are made between those who are permanently and those who are temporarily polluted by their contact with death. Admittedly the Cantonese example is an extreme one, since Cantonese funeral specialists are strictly segregated from the rest of the community after the funeral ceremony and not permitted to return to the village until they are required for the next funeral. Nevertheless, the general picture may be suggestive for the Roman situation. There are some residual indications at Rome of similar ideas about those who approach a corpse and how such people were viewed by the rest of society.

An embalmer (*pollinctor*) was sometimes hired to prepare the body of the deceased for burial. How often this preparation fell to such funeral specialists cannot be ascertained from the available evidence. Poor families may have been prevented from using the services of a *pollinctor* by expense. The preparation of the body could be considered to create a situation filled with ambivalence. The heir was expected to have supervisory control over all the funeral arrangements. On the one hand, as a question of *pietas* the family, and in particular the heir, were expected to be directly involved in preparation of the body for burial and to show appropriate respect for the deceased. On the other, their role had the effect of exposing both family and heir to some measure of pollution, even if they did not actually handle the corpse. In due course their actions would require acts of purification. It may be that the washing of the body was normally performed by the wife or mother of the deceased, as was the case in Greece, thus keeping this personal act in family hands (Garland 1985: ch. 3).

Even if the *pollinctor* did not always wash the body, he probably was employed to perfume it. The principle aim of this was to prevent the rapid decomposition of the body. Miscellaneous elements including salt, honey and myrrh were used as preservatives. The Law of the Twelve Tables prohibited the use of myrrh and slave labour for this purpose, but the regulations appear to have been widely ignored (Cic. *Leg.* 2.24). A *pollinctor* was frequently employed and would be a slave who would become ritually polluted as a result of his contact with the body of the deceased; it would seem that his very lowly status (*infamis*, i.e. disgraced) should be explained in terms of this contact (cf. Bodel, in this volume).

The prohibition under the Law of the Twelve Tables partly related to the great expense of myrrh which was obtained from Carthaginian sources. Doubtless the measure had sumptuary intent, and may be seen as an attempt to prevent excessive amounts from being expended on funerals. Cicero tells us that these restrictions were an inheritance from the laws of Solon (Cic. *Leg.* 2.23ff; cf. Plut. *Sol.* 21). In the empire embalming came to be associated with Egyptianising tendencies, and sources tend to be hostile (Counts 1996: 189–202). Restrictions on embalming can thus be traced to early legislation on Roman funerals. Other requirements included a stipulation that the pyre should not be smoothed over with an axe, and that expense was to be limited to three veils, a purple tunic and ten flautists. Garland has pointed out, in relation to Greek funerals, that attempts to reduce expenditures on funerals are closely related to the fact that 'funerary and post-funerary rituals tend to promote divisiveness and factionalism among the citizen body, by providing rival aristocratic kin-groups or *gene* with an opportunity to further their sectarian interests to the detriment of society as a whole' (Garland 1989: 1–15). The failure at Rome to reduce aristocratic display at funerals can be explained in terms of the very different and undemocratic direction taken by political life in that city.

Once the body was prepared other professionals may have been employed to assist with the funeral. A *dissignator* (undertaker) seems originally to have been an official who guided spectators to their seats in the theatre (e.g. *CIL* VI 373, 1074, 1955, 2223, 8846, 32332; Weaver 1972: 82 n. 6). Perhaps the term first came to be applied to the undertaker when funerary games were celebrated in honour of the distinguished dead. Indeed it has been suggested that the *dissignator* is only found at aristocratic funerals as an organiser of the procession (Toynbee 1971: 45; Flower 1996: 116). He would be accompanied by assistants dressed in black (Hor. *Ep.* 1.7.6). Nevertheless, the term seems to be used interchangeably with that of *libitinarius* by Seneca to designate undertakers as a class. The term *libitinarius* relates to the role of Libitina in keeping a record of deaths (Suet. *Nero* 39). Seneca pours scorn on inheritance-hunters (*captatores*), and alleges that *dissignatores* and *libitinarii* are in fact less disgusting since they do not pray for the destruction of their immediate acquaintance (Sen. *Ben.* 6.38.4). This vituperation takes on greater significance when the unmentionably lowly status of the undertakers is borne in mind (Gardner 1993: 130ff; Bodel, in this volume).

Our best evidence on funeral professionals is not from Rome, but from Puteoli and Cumae, and consists of two similar municipal laws about local arrangements for conducting burials and executions, both public and private (*AE* 1971 88, 89). They have been discussed recently and comprehensively by John Bodel (1994; and in this volume). These laws relating to Libitina (*leges libitinariae*) provide guidelines for the contractor and his employees, and include restrictions on their place of residence. I cite here the relevant section of the law from Puteoli (*AE* 1971 88):

> The workers who are to provide this service are not to live on this side of the tower where the grove of Libitina is today and are to bathe after the first hour of the night. They are not to enter the town except for the purpose of carrying off and relocating corpses, or exacting punishment. While and as often as in this way one of them comes to, enters, or is in the town he should have on his head a red cap.[2]
>
> (Bodel 1994: 72–80; Gardner and Wiedemann 1991: 24–6)

The local grove of Libitina at Puteoli may have been modelled on its counterpart in Rome, and the legislation of the two towns may have been similar. Of course we cannot confirm that the residence restriction mentioned here is based on anything more than considerations of hygiene, but the Chinese parallel may be suggestive. Very careful segregation and stigmatisation of the corpse-handlers in Cantonese funerals is indicative of their despised and polluted state, and is related not just to hygiene but also to ideas of spiritual pollution (Watson 1988: 124–6). At Puteoli segregation through distinctive dress and time of bathing shows at the very least entrenched ideas about avoidance of this group.

The term for a grave-digger was *fossor* and appears in a Republican context in a well-known poem of Catullus (22.9–11):

> When you read this, that fine and witty Suffenus seems once more to be a goat herd or grave digger [fossor]; so much does he shrink away and change.

Here *fossor* is used as a term of abuse, apparently with no stronger force than to indicate lowly social status; Suffenus is uncouth and clumsy (*OLD* s.v. 'fossor'). Catullus doubtless chose the term because of its ill-omened associations. Although the evidence is insufficient to show that the grave-digger had such lowly status because of his potential to pollute, this might be a reasonable inference. Those employed to burn corpses (*ustores*) are also mentioned with hostility by both Catullus and Martial as an example of persons engaged in a degrading occupation (Cat. 59.5; Mart. 3.93.26–7). Both authors introduce the polluted and lowly *ustor* as a disgusting figure inappropriate to a civilised context.

The stigma of the funeral trade can thus be seen to have had a considerable impact on the lives of funerary workers in Rome which parallels, at least in part, the Cantonese evidence. Elsewhere in this volume Bodel explores the nature and reasons for these stigmas in more detail, and also notes some similarities between the treatment of undertakers and executioners. The *carnifex* (executioner) was considered a disgrace (*infamis*) and could not live in the city (Plaut. *Pseud.* 332; Cic. *Pro C. Rab.* 5.15; David 1984: 144). Catullus uses him as an extreme example of baseness (97.12). He was not a respectable part of the life of the city – shunned for example by the Vestal Cornelia as a proof of her chastity under Domitian (Plin. *Ep.* 4.11; cf. Juv. 8.175). Unlike the tribune who was not polluted by those he condemned to death, the executioner was a marginal figure in the world of the living.

These examples from Rome of death-pollution associated with both the corpse and those in proximity to it do not show the extreme attitudes of the Chinese context, but may give a pale reflection of the taboos of a bygone era. Pollution after a death resulted in some level of avoidance of the bereaved family. Priests and especially the priest of Jupiter seem to have been subject to special taboos. Those providing funerary services were undoubtedly shunned by polite society, and may have been felt to have been engaged not merely in a distasteful activity, but in one which conferred on them some level of pollution. There are considerable difficulties in defining the nature of the shunning. Physical, hygienic or spiritual considerations may each have had a part to play, and it is far from certain if contemporary Romans were totally aware of reasons for the low repute of funeral workers.

The rituals of transition

In this section, the aim is to outline the main features of rituals from the deathbed scene to the tomb, with an eye to those rituals which seem to reflect concerns over death-pollution. In addition there is an examination of the subsequent purification of the family and the extent to which the rites of incineration and burial satisfied hygienic requirements and concerns over the fate of the soul.

Hired musicians and the deathbed scene

The moment of death is characteristically marked by a final sigh or kiss, and literary sources place much emphasis on famous last words. The case of Augustus exemplifies both of these phenomena, since he both kisses Livia and bids her remember whose wife she has been (Suet. *Aug.* 99). In Seneca's *Consolatio ad Marciam* the fact that Octavia was deprived of the chance to savour her son's last kiss and to enjoy his final words through Drusus' death on the Rhine is seen as a dislocation of the desired pattern (Sen. *Cons. Ad Marc.* 3.1–2). The Epicurean Aufidius Bassus hoped that there would be no pain in his final breath, and took consolation in the very brevity of that last sigh. In accordance with Epicurean belief he imagined that all pain for him would end with that last pain. He had anticipated the easy departure of his soul since he was an old man, and he believed it was thus located close to the door of his lips (Sen. *Ep.* 30.14ff.).

The deathbed may not have been, however, a very peaceful place. In some instances, when a Roman is about to die or has just died, musicians appear to be present (Toynbee 1971: pl. 11; Ariès 1981: 95–139). It appears that their presence always playing loud instruments – the trumpet, the tambourine – is intended to give warning of the existence of a funeral, and also to assist in stage-managing critical elements of the ritual. In Cantonese ritual the approach of the corpse-handlers is announced by a loud burst of piping to enable family members to avert their eyes from the polluting sight of the wrapping-up of the body (Watson 1988: 124–5). While it appears that a less strict view was taken of the potential pollution from undertakers at Rome, it can be imagined that the role of musicians was still to alert family members and the outside world to the dangers of pollution. John Bodel has suggested that the headquarters of the association of flute-players was located just outside the Esquiline Gate near the grove of Libitina (*lucus Libitinae*) (Bodel 1994: 50; Coarelli 1996a). Perhaps the Romans considered them as polluted as a result of their role in the death-ritual, thus explaining the location of their headquarters outside the mainstream activities of the city.

In the Cantonese context the musicians represent the male counterpart of the high-pitched female keening which intimated a death (Johnson 1988: 135–63). In either case the main purpose of the procedure is public announcement of the death. Roman representations of death often include musicians as well as female mourners; the best example is the lying-in-state (*collocatio*) depicted on the relief of the Haterii from the Via Labicana in Rome (now in the Vatican), where the mourners are depicted beating their breasts, and it may be assumed that there was accompanying lamentation (Cuq 1881: 1391; Toynbee 1971: 44–5 with pl. 9). No literary source identifies a precise role for musicians at Roman funerals. Anthropologists have noticed that the use of noisy instruments at funerals is widespread in diverse cultural contexts, and suggest that there is a connection between percussion and transition (Needham 1967: 606–14). Although these discussions tend to centre on drums in an African context, where comparison has been made between the drumbeat and the heartbeat and rhythm of life, it can be appreciated that the aim of piping can also be related to the marking of temporal change (Huntington and Metcalf 1979: 46–50).

In relation to religious ritual a piper was employed by the Romans when a chief magistrate was uttering a prayer to prevent anything but the words of the prayer from being heard. The same purpose has been thought to lie behind the use of pipes at the funeral, that is to prevent the dying man from hearing imprecations which could harm him, or to counteract the effect of those who wanted to vow his soul to the infernal divinities (Pliny *NH* 28.11; Tac. *Ann.* 2.69).

The conclamatio

When death occurred the eyes of the deceased would be closed, perhaps by a close female relative. In the case of parents their eyes would commonly be closed by their offspring. Next would be the ritual of calling on the deceased, known as *conclamatio* (Servius on Verg. *Aen.* 6.218). This procedure was continued until such time as the body was carried off for cremation or burial. By early imperial times the ritual significance of this act appears to be in decline. It represents an appeal to the soul of the deceased to indicate that events are in train for a decent burial (*iusta sepultura*), and is also a check on whether death has in fact taken place. The *conclamatio* is continued throughout the funeral ritual until the burial (*humatio*) when a final adieu is said to the deceased and a wish is expressed that the earth be light upon him (Toynbee 1971: 44 and pl. 10).

Preparing the body

After the *conclamatio* the body is taken down from the bed, rested on its knees, as if to see whether life has abandoned it, then laid on the ground, washed in warm water and perfumed to prevent rapid decomposition (Servius on Verg. *Aen.* 6.218). As pointed out above, by the late Republic this operation was commonly performed by the *pollinctor*. The process of washing the body in warm water might also be an effective method of ensuring that the subject was no longer alive.

The body thus prepared would be dressed in a toga even in an age when it was more normal for citizens to wear the tunic. Juvenal could say that nobody in his time wore the toga except after death (Juv. 3.171). Generally a white toga was used. In cases of extreme poverty the corpse would be wrapped in a piece of black cloth. But the emphasis was on display, and the aim was to provide expensive cloth and to emblazon the body with the insignia of the highest public functions attained, especially magistracies. Livy suggests that with the advent of the Gauls in 390 BC senators prepared for death by donning their finery (Livy 5.41). This could include crowns gained during life either in public games or through bravery. Christian writers later complained that this made the corpse into a sort of idol (Tert. *De Coron.* 10). By contrast, those attending a funeral would dress in black (Flower 1996: 102), and commonly disfigure themselves by covering their hair with ashes as a token of mourning (Catullus 64.349–51; Verg. *Aen.* 10.844, 12.611).

Exposition

According to Pollux (writing in the age of the Antonines) the aim of exposition was to show that the death had not been caused by an act of violence (Pollux 8.1). As an essential part of the process leading to the funeral itself, the body would be laid out on a prepared funerary couch in the *atrium* of the house with its feet facing the front door. What happened to those who had no *atrium* remains obscure, but the idea was to display the body in a prominent place in the house. Apparently it was the duty of close relatives themselves to place the corpse on the couch on which it was to be exposed. Perfumes would be burned in an incense burner (*acerra*) and flowers representing the fragility of life would be scattered around the bed. The clearest iconographic example of exposition or lying in state (known as *collocatio*) is to be found on the relief of the Haterii from the Lateran collection in the Vatican, mentioned above (Toynbee 1971: pl. 9). The subject is the exposition of a woman (probably herself a freedwoman of some wealth) who is surrounded by burning torches, attendants and flute-players (*praeficae* and *tibicines*). There are also three women wearing the cap of freedom, the *pileus*, presumed to be slave women freed under her will (Giuliano 1968: 449–82; Coarelli 1979: 255–69; Flower 1996: 93–4).

*Carrying out the body (*efferre, foras ferre*) and the* laudatio

The body was next removed from the house of death and a group of friends were invited to follow the convoy: hence the name of this segment of the ceremony, *exsequiae*. Invitation was usually made by a freedman who invited the parents and friends of the deceased to come to the obsequies (Varro *Rust.*

1.69). This often occurred on the day following the decease, provided it was not a public holiday (Cic. *Clu.* 9; Ter. *An.* 105ff.).

The splendour of the cortège would depend greatly on the status of the deceased, as would its destination. For a public funeral the procession would proceed to the Forum Romanum for the funeral laudation (*laudatio funebris*) (Vollmer 1891: 445–528; Kierdorf 1980), but it is probable that most funerals were conducted in a less public manner at the graveside. There is doubt, for example, over whether the *laudatio Turiae* (*EJ*^{2} 357) was delivered from the rostra in the Forum Romanum, and it is more likely that this type of commemoration was conducted privately at the tomb (Horsfall 1983: 85–98).

Mimicry is an extremely prominent element in Roman funerals. A traditional accompaniment for the entourage at the last rites of the illustrious was a satyr dance performed by hired actors (the *sicinnis*), which Dionysius of Halicarnassus believed to be of Greek origin (Dion. Hal. *Ant. Rom.* 7.72). The role of these satyrs was to ridicule the person who in other ways was being accorded the highest respect, and Dionysius notes that in like manner, on the occasion of a triumph soldiers dressed as satyrs were allowed to ridicule the *triumphator*. Processions at funerals and triumphs have several important similarities; although work on the triumph has until recently tended to emphasise Etruscan influence (Bonfante Warren 1970: 49–66; Versnel 1970: 115–29), the importance of Hellenistic elements is now being recognised (Flower 1996: 105–9). One highly important aspect of the triumph was the ritual purification of the general (Bonfante Warren 1970: 52–3). His performance of a ritual act of cleansing (the *lustratio*) was critical to the triumphal ceremony and may be seen as a link with overall objectives of the funerary rites. Whatever their origin, ludicrous elements in Roman processions such as the satyr dance seem to have had an apotropaic purpose; they were intended to avert the evil eye. This is clearest in the case of the triumph when the *triumphator* had to be reminded of his mortality by a slave: 'look behind you and remember that you are a man' (*respice post te! Hominem te memento*: Tert. *Apol.* 33; cf. Zon. 7.21).

Actors wearing wax *imagines* were also prominent in the funeral rituals (Lindsay 1996: 271–85). Polybius explains the function of the *imagines* (Polyb. 6.53–4). When a significant member of a prominent family died, actors who bore a striking resemblance to the subject's ancestors in stature and gait wore the masks in the funeral procession. This macabre mimicry was enhanced by the colours applied to the mask to accentuate its verisimilitude. Furthermore the actors would be clothed as befitted the rank of the highest office held by the ancestor, and on reaching the rostra would sit on the curule chairs appropriate to them. The actual colouring of the masks has attracted attention, since it was felt that this too might be an element held in common with the triumph. A triumphing general was painted with a red dye (*minium*), as was Jupiter Capitolinus himself, for reasons which have been much discussed, and Bömer tentatively suggested that the ancestral masks might also have been coloured in this way. It is certainly interesting to note that red colour has been discovered on other funerary items such as skeletons, urns and coffins, and particularly skulls from pre Indo-European tombs in Italy, and we might expect to find some trace of the employment of red dye or the use of masks in later practice (Bömer 1943: 104ff.). However, our information on the significance of colouring and the role of the masks is incomplete, and the idea that anything other than verisimilitude was the aim has recently been rejected by Flower (Flower 1996: 109–15). Nevertheless, it should be emphasised that the whole ritual appears not only to be highly theatrical, but also a response to the process of transition which the corpse is undergoing. The corpse is moving from the world of the living to join the ancestral group who are being impersonated by the actors. The activities at the funeral intentionally create a liminal performance to commemorate the event. Rites of passage commonly do involve elaborate rituals, although as here it is often not possible to separate symbolic from merely commemorative acts.

Suetonius provides us with an account of the chief buffoon (*archmimus*) Favor, who was hired to provide this traditional mimicry at the funeral of Vespasian. As Polybius had done earlier, Suetonius emphasises that the mime was to imitate the words and idiosyncrasies of the deceased. Favor exceeded his brief, wittily mimicking the notorious parsimony of Vespasian (Suet. *Vesp.* 19). By this stage it seems that the ritual has been resuscitated as a venerable antique, and mimicry is not prominent in other imperial funerals about which we are well informed (Price 1987: 56–105; Arce 1990).

From the laudatio *to the tomb*

After the commemorative speech the corpse would be transferred from the couch on which it had been displayed into a sort of wooden coffin consisting of an open bier (*capulus*) (Apul. *Met.* 4.18; Festus-Paulus 53L s.v. 'capulum'; Serv. *ad Aen.* 11.64; Non. Marc. 19–31). In cases of violent death, and perhaps also when decomposition had set in, the face would be veiled (Vell. 2.4.6; Dio 61.7). This coffin would be transferred onto a stretcher (*feretrum*) and carried in the manner of a litter, as can be seen particularly clearly on the well-known relief from Amiternum (Toynbee 1971: pl. 11). For the impoverished the stretcher and coffin would be combined and went under the name of *sandapila*. Domitian's assassination and his subsequently damned reputation (*damnatio memoriae*) explain how a person of imperial rank could suffer the humiliation of a *sandapila* (Suet. *Dom.* 17; cf. Mart. 10.5.9; on *damnatio memoriae* see Pailler and Sablayrolles 1994: 11–55). This disgrace had to be dealt with expeditiously for the sake of future stability, and thus Domitian's body was removed quickly and subjected to very summary treatment.

The stretcher would then be carried at shoulder height by six or eight bearers in the case of a litter, four in the case of a *sandapila* (Mart. 2.81.1, 8.75.9). Sons, close relatives or heirs considered it an honour to be called upon (Serv. *ad Aen.* 6.222). An illustration of this is the funeral of Metellus Macedonicus, who was carried by his four sons, of whom one was praetor and the others had been censors or consuls (Pliny *NH* 7.44; Val. Max. 7.1.1). Sometimes it seems that those whom the deceased had supported and helped would volunteer for the task. At this juncture slaves who were to be given their liberty under his will would frequently offer their services (Pliny *NH* 18.16; Plut. *Aem.* 39; Pers. *Sat.* 3.103–6). In the case of the poor or insignificant, there existed pall-bearers called *vespillones* who charged for this service. They were also called *sandapilarii* because of the type of coffin they would transport. In the age of Constantine the emperor set up a corporation of *lecticarii* at Constantinople, and they would transport corpses of the indigent free of charge (Nov. Just. 43, 59). This practice may have been modelled on early imperial benefactions.

Purification of the family

The process of transition, alluded to above, had an impact not merely on the deceased, but also on the mourners. Both the family and the house of death faced rituals of purification, a cleansing which was both moral and physical. The rituals recorded in sources such as Cicero and Festus-Paulus seem archaic.[3] It is difficult to judge how long they persisted, but by the second century AD they seem to have been fossils.

Responsibilty for the ritual cleansing fell to the *euerriator* who corresponded to the heir, according to Festus-Paulus (Festus-Paulus 68L s.v. 'euerriator'). No doubt this responsibility under the influence of pontifical law was extended to whoever acquired control of the *sacra*, that is maintenance of the cult of the family. The term *euerriator* was derived from *extra uerrere*, to sweep out. The ritual had serious repercussions since failure to sweep out the house of death, or any inadequacy in the operation, was thought to be expiated by death. A special type of broom had to be employed for the purging (Festus-Paulus loc. cit.). It seems that the cleaning took place immediately after the removal of the body for burial.

Chronology at this stage in the ritual cleansing causes some problems (Lindsay 1998: 72–3). There were days of rest and mourning after a death known as the *feriae denicales* (Cic. *Leg.* 2.22.55; Festus-Paulus 61L s.v. 'denicales feriae'); these followed the funeral and were brought to an end by the sacrifice on the ninth day (*novemdial sacrificium*). Cicero has few ideas about the etymology of the term *feriae denicales* or the precise significance of the institution, although he situates the mourning in the context of respect for the ancestral rites of the individual, and underlines the presence of ritual elements. It is not immediately apparent whether the *novemdial sacrificium* was the same as the *silicernium*; this latter was a funerary meal which occurred at the tomb itself, and consisted of a sausage. This food may originally have had a ritual significance (Festus-Paulus 377L; see Lindsay 1998: 72). However, it is plausible to imagine that the *silicernium* occurred at the time of burial and before the *feriae denicales*. The *novemdial* can then be associated with a later stage of purification known from Cicero's account, the sacrifice of wethers to the Lar, and can be thought of as a conclusion to the period of mourning known as the *feriae denicales*. In the interim many types of activity were taboo and it seems such matters were closely monitored by the pontiffs (Aul. Gell. *NA* 16.4.4; Columella *Rust.* 2.21).

At the funerary meal known as the *silicernium* (Festus-Paulus 377L), the heir seems to have been obliged to sacrifice a sow to Ceres (or possibly to Ceres and Tellus) under a ritual which was to take place in the presence of the deceased (*porca praesentanea*) (Le Bonniec 1958: 93ff.). This sacrifice is an obscurity only recorded by Veranius Flaccus, a contemporary of Varro (and reported by Festus-Paulus 296L).

As far as can be ascertained the *porca praesentanea* was an obligatory sacrifice of a sow in the presence of the corpse in every instance of decease. It represents an expiation (*piaculum*) undertaken to cleanse the pollution of the *familia*, and can be contrasted with the *porca praecidanea*, a preliminary sow sacrifice which would only be offered in cases where some omission or error had occurred. The menu for the funeral feast was fixed by usage: eggs, vegetables, beans, lentils and salt (Juv. 5.85; Lucian *Catapl.* 7; Tac. *Ann.* 6.5; Plut. *Quaest. conv.* VII; Hor. *Serm.* 2.6.63; Plut. *Crass.* 19). What is notable about this occasion is how the role of the funerary rite as an event centred, at least partially, on the deceased could be subverted. In some cases an heir irritated by the deceased for some reason would abstain from inviting those who assisted at the funeral (Pers. *Sat.* 6.33). The occasion could also develop into a debauch, despite a provision of the Law of the Twelve Tables prohibiting continuous drinking rounds (*circumpotatio*) (Athen. 8.34; Cic. *Leg.* 2.24). In theory the deceased was not forgotten; food and wine were placed on his tomb. This provided a temptation for the indigent, who would undergo pollution if they ate this food (Tibull. 1.5.53). Plautus calls them grave-robbers (*bustirapi*: Pseudol. 348).

On return from the funeral those who had participated in the interment had to be purified with fire and water. This stage in the cleansing is called the *suffitio* (Festus-Paulus 3L s.v. 'aqua et igni'). The ritual involved using a laurel branch to sprinkle water on the participants, after which they were made to pass under the fire. An older term related to this ritual, the precise significance of which is lost, is the word *exfir* (Festus-Paulus 69L s.v. 'exfir'). The use of the laurel to purge the pollution of death is also found in association with the triumph (Festus-Paulus 104L s.v. 'laureati'). Festus-Paulus uses the past tense in his description of the *suffitio*, as though it was no longer carried out in his own time.

Burial: incineration versus inhumation

Incineration as a rite can be thought of as an inherently tidier and more hygienic method of disposing of a corpse than inhumation, which ultimately involves decay and decomposition. Although practical considerations had a part in deciding on the rites employed for burial in ancient Rome, it will also be appropriate to investigate how different rites for disposal of the body were viewed in relation to questions of pollution and its subsequent purification. Specifically the central issue here is how effective each rite was considered in the settling of the spirit world.

Although both incineration and inhumation co-existed at Rome from the beginnings of the city, it would seem that incineration soon came to prominence, so much so that the *gens Cornelia* became celebrated for its persistence in using inhumation. Even the fact that the Law of the Twelve Tables cites the two modes of burial may only be a homage to pontifical tradition. In the case of incineration, the pontiffs continued to insist on symbolic inhumations. These were the *iniectio glebae* which involved the casting of a little earth over the mortal remains even after a cremation, and the burial of the *os resectum*, a small piece of the corpse retained for subsequent burial (De Visscher 1963: 8–9, 26). Pontifical law thus appears to be rooted in inhumation. The purpose of the symbolic burials was related to pontifical concern that the deceased should be assured a *locus religiosus* (a respected place of burial).

If the burial was inadequately executed it was thought that the soul of the deceased could return to haunt the living. Thus Caligula's ghost was said to haunt the Lamian gardens until a proper funeral was organised by his sisters on their return from exile (Suet. *Calig.* 59). His initial cremation had been incomplete, and the body was not properly buried. This resulted in a pollution which was believed to have been expiated when his sisters completed the funeral rites.

Roman beliefs about the resting-place of the soul were varied. The Stoic philosophers limited the duration of the soul's stay in the tomb by reference to the decomposition of the body (Serv. *ad Aen.* 3.68). In contrast under incineration it was believed that the spirits of the dead (*Manes*) departed to the underworld (*Orcus*) and only continued a life there as an undifferentiated group. The status of an individual ghost within this group depended not on his own behaviour during lifetime but on the behaviour of the living in regard to their cult (De Visscher 1963: 28–31).

In summary, the rituals of transition from deathbed to grave were complex. Music which was played at the deathbed may have originally had a symbolic function. There were expectations that close kin would be involved in the closing of the eyes on death, and the ritual calling on the deceased was intended both to ensure that death had occurred, and to advertise the fact that proper burial of the subject was in train. The body was prepared by family, or sometimes an embalmer, and some level of pollution was considered to fall both on those who were involved in the funeral and on the house of death. The exposition of the body seems to have links with Etruscan customs, and in the case of aristocrats display in the atrium becomes an opportunity to publicise status. This was reinforced by dressing the corpse in finery, and by the splendour of the theatrical display in the procession on the way to the rostra. Hellenistic processions influenced the ritual, but the funeral procession still shows signs of remaining an important rite of transition in the late Republic. By the imperial period decline has set in and emphasis seems to be on the theatre of the occasion rather than its ritual significance. After the removal of the body for burial, the family had to engage in acts of purification which reflected the need for both physical and spiritual cleansing in the aftermath of the ill-omened event. Both cremation and inhumation were methods of disposing of the body which satisfied the hygienic and spiritual requirements of the occasion. Acts of cleansing which may originally have been understood in a religious sense appear to have declined and been little understood in the imperial period.

Legislation on the location of graves at Rome

In this final section the limited evidence on legislation concerned with the siting of graves is examined. The aim is to try to identify the rationale behind the rules relating to the exclusion of graves from certain areas, and to attempt to establish whether hygienic or spiritual issues are most prominent.

Legislative enactments on the location of graves existed from an early period. Nothing concrete is known of the period prior to the Laws of the Twelve Tables. According to Dionysius of Halicarnassus and Servius, in the earliest days of the city Romans buried their dead within the bounds of the city (Dion. Hal. *Ant. Rom.* 3.1; Serv. *ad Aen.* 11.206), and even in their houses (Serv. *ad Aen.* 5.64, 6.152). Cicero, however, thought that only exceptional individuals had ever been buried in the city. Thus he relates that Poblicola and Tubertus were allowed burial within the city on grounds of merit in the period before the matter was legally regulated, while Gaius Fabricius had obtained the same concession after the Laws of the Twelve Tables were in operation (Cic. *Leg.* 2.23.58).

Cicero believed that it was Decemviral law which first prohibited burial or cremation of corpses within the sacred boundary of the city (the *pomerium*, on which see Labrousse 1937: 165–99; Boatwright 1986: 13–27; Syme 1983: 131ff.). Cicero attributes this prohibition to a fear of fires, plausible in the case of cremation, but not so for inhumation (Cic. *Leg.* 2.23.58; Bodel 1994: 33). His attitude is however revealing, because it shows that by the late Republic it was practical considerations rather than superstition which determined practice in relation to such matters. Interestingly, Isidore of

Seville alleges the prohibition was based on fear of the putrid smell emanating from corpses (Isidor. *Orig.* 15.11). Cuq concludes that the Decemvirs had been influenced by the doctrine of Heraclitus that a corpse is no more than a pile of refuse to be disposed of like manure (Cuq 1881: s.v. 'funus' 1392). This may be thought of as additional evidence that practical factors such as questions of hygiene had lasting importance in ancient thinking about the disposal of corpses.

As pointed out by Atticus, whatever the reason for excluding corpses from the city, the prohibition had not lasted to his own time, since it had become customary to bury distinguished citizens within the city (Cic. *Leg.* 2.23.58). Moreover, Cicero says, as noted above, that even before the Law of the Twelve Tables some distinguished citizens were permitted burial within the city; what pontifical law added was prohibition of burial on public ground. The reason for this was that the pontiffs felt it inappropriate for private and public rites to be intermingled. Cicero gives a specific example of how in the case of the temple of Honour outside the Colline gate private graves had to be removed to enable the public cult of Honour to be established (Cic. *Leg.* 2.23.58). This again shows that practicalities were more important than superstitious dread – graves were not considered to be of necessity permanently inviolable.

The prohibition under the Law of the Twelve Tables was never applied to children under four days old, who would be buried *sub grundo*, that is under the porch facing into the courtyard (Ful. *Serm. ant.* 560.13). But for others, the prohibition was repeatedly confirmed, for example by a decree of the senate in the consulate of Duillius in 260 BC (Serv. *Ad aen.* 11.206). A similar provision is also to be found in the colony of Genetiva Julia (44 BC), which established a financial penalty of 5,000HS (*CIL* XII 594 = *ILS* 6087). A senatorial decree of 38 BC prohibited the burning of bodies within two miles of Rome (Dio 48.43.3). The distance from the city has been thought to show that the primary concern was not an infringement of the *pomerium*, but rather public safety (Bodel 1994: 33).

In the second century AD, Hadrian, in a rescript, prescribed a pecuniary penalty for those who contravened the restriction on burial within two miles of the city, as well as for the magistrates who turned a blind eye. Moreover, the land concerned was to be confiscated, and the corpse exhumed and buried elsewhere (Ulp. *Digest* 47.12.3.5). Could this rescript apply not only at Rome but also in those municipalities which permitted burial within the city limits? In reality rescripts seem to have had a limited impact outside Rome. Under Antoninus Pius there was a further attempt to enforce the rule (*SHA Ant. Pius* 12). Eventually Diocletian confirmed the opinion of Ulpian, and that imperial rescripts were to apply to all municipalities (Cod. *Iust.* 3.44.12).

The rule was gradually broken down in the late Empire under the impact of Christianity, which encouraged the conservation of the relics of saints within cities. The earliest moves in this direction took place in Constantinople, and the privilege was gradually extended to emperors, bishops and other notables. Theodosius I in AD 381 tried to turn the clock back (Cod. *Theod.* 9.17.6), and it was not until the ninth century that the emperor Leo finally officially removed the interdiction on burial within the city which had been legally controlled since the time of the Twelve Tables (Cuq 1881: s.v. 'funus' 1393).

John Bodel's recent study of the *Lex Lucerina* has suggested that the primary concern in legislation on the location of graves is with considerations of hygiene and not religious dread (Bodel 1994: 33). We need not assume that Romans appreciated the concept of contagion to accept that this became the dominant reason for locating cemeteries outside cities. It is only too clear that sanitation was a major and persistent problem in urban centres (Scobie 1986: 399–433). It will certainly have been a major consideration, even if in some quarters fear of rampant souls reinforced the desirability of excluding corpses from the city.

As the city expanded, areas formerly reserved for burials became incorporated within the *pomerium* (Patterson, in this volume). Since this must often have involved the removal of old tombs, a general question of great importance is how long a grave remained an object of veneration before it became possible to ignore its religious associations. Roman views of the soul will have had an impact in this area, as will the notion of a tomb as a status indicator for an individual family. Conclusions are hard to reach through scarcity of evidence, but the following points may be suggestive.

We can note some formulas, common in epitaphs, which show a reaction against the hereditary principle for tombs. In general family tombs under pontifical law fell automatically to the agnatic descendants whether or not they were heirs. A different principle was involved with hereditary tombs, which could clearly move outside the family group. Under the pontifical law, the *sacra*, particularly in cases of intestacy, might well fall outside the family group. Some testators seem to have disliked the pontifical rules to the extent of excluding these 'heirs' from burial. These are probably cases where a will exists and the testator already knows that an heir of his own blood (i.e. an agnatic heir) will not follow him. These cases are indicated on tombs by the inscription HMHNS: *Hoc monumentum heredem non sequetur* (this monument shall not fall to the share of the heir) or HMHENS: *Hoc monumentum heredem exterum non sequetur* (this monument shall not fall to the share of an heir who is an outsider). In the former case there is some possibility that the testator does not wish an heir even of his own blood to inherit the tomb. This could be seen as a reaction to the increased importance attached to the memorial function of the tomb. In the late Republic the shrine that Cicero planned for his daughter Tullia, thought to have been located on the site of the Farnesina, was intended as an individual memorial (Lavagne 1987: 160–2). The early imperial Petronius envisages the freedman Trimalchio demanding a personalised memorial in a passage that exemplifies the ambitions of the social climbing freedman. All the emphasis is on the preservation of a personal domain after death, surrounded by gardens and vineyards, tended by a freedman custodian, and including provision for suitable memorial dinners, for which he has provided through a foundation (Petron. *Sat.* 71.6–9; Purcell 1987: 25). The public orientation of this display shows how far an early imperial tomb is entrenched in the lives of the living.

Conclusion

Defining death-pollution, both the way in which it operated and the way in which it was understood, is a complex process. On the one hand it appears that in the Roman world certain taboos surrounded the corpse and the bereaved. A death in a Roman family resulted in a level of avoidance of family members during the period of direct contact with the corpse and subsequent mourning; rites of purification and sacrifice had to be performed by the family to placate the dead and to remove pollution; priests, particularly the priest of Jupiter, are said to have had a special concern to avoid the corpse; and undertakers were despised and reviled at Rome, partly because they were of low status but also because they were in some ways polluted by the nature of their work. On the other hand the corpse and family were treated with respect. Death could provide opportunities for celebration and display; the body could be decked in fineries, exhibited in the house, carried in public procession, praised extravagantly and finally buried in style. A death was not only about loss, grief and appropriate rituals, it was also about status and the continuity of the family. This underlines how events surrounding death were not controlled purely by religious dread and fear but were often motivated by more mundane practical concerns.

Indeed for many aspects of death-pollution itself it is impossible to isolate spiritual or religious rationale from more practical aspects, such as hygiene. In the case of undertakers, for example, it is hard to ascertain whether these workers were shunned due to distaste for the work they performed or because of specific issues relating to hygienic or even spiritual pollution. Often we are confronted by uncertainties and ambiguities in the available sources. The reason why some rituals were performed and some objects, people and actions were regarded as polluted was not always fully understood. In addition attitudes and beliefs changed across time, making some rituals anachronistic if not irrelevant. Indeed a recurring problem is the difficulty of knowing what people did actually believe about the fate of the dead and thus death-pollution. Isolating and identifying elements such as tradition, superstition and religion, plus aspects such as social status and education, which would have all influenced how people viewed death and the dead, frequently eludes us.

A good illustration of all these difficulties is provided by the legislation concerning the location of graves. The main authorities seem to have had an incomplete understanding of why tombs and the dead were excluded from the city and the relative roles of religion, hygiene and safety. On one level this suggests that these elements were entwined and mutually enforcing; merging together as a result of an evolutionary process. Nevertheless the regulations themselves from the late Republic and early imperial period, concerning cremation and burial, suggest that matters of hygiene and safety did come to the fore. In addition the growth of the memorial function of tombs shows that increasingly they came to be regarded as status indicators rather than objects of religious veneration. This is not to suggest that religion ceased to play a role in influencing the behaviour surrounding death, but in a materialistic and status-conscious world, distinctions between different types of pollution were perhaps easily and conveniently blurred.

NOTES

1 I have included evidence from the fourth-century Vergilian commentator Servius since his focus is antiquarian.

2 *oper(ae) quae at eam r(em) praeparat(ae) er(unt) ne intra turrem ubi hodie lucus est Libit(inae) habitent laventurve ab h(ora) I/noctis neve veniant in oppid(um) nisi mortui tollend(i) conlocand(i)ve aut supplic(i) sumend(i) c(ausa); dum ita/quis eor(um) veniat quotiens oppid(um) intrab(it) in oppid(o)ve erit ut pilleum color(atum) in capit(e) habea{nt}.*

3 The value and methods of Festus-Paulus have recently been explored in Grandazzi 1991: 101–23.

BIBLIOGRAPHY

Adcock, F. (1927) 'The Attacks on the Friends of Pericles', *Cambridge Ancient History*, vol. 5, Cambridge: Cambridge University Press, 477–80.

Aigner, H. (1988) 'Zur gesellschaftlichen Stellung von Henkern, Gladiatoren und Berufsathleten', in I. Weiler (ed.), *Soziale Randgruppen und Aussenseiter im Altertum*, Graz: Leykam, 201–20.

Allara, A. (1995) '*Corpus* et *cadaver*, la "gestion" d'un nouveau corpus', in F. Hinard (ed.), *La mort au quotidien dans le monde Romain*, Paris: De Boccard, 69–79.

André, J.-M. (1980) 'La notion de Pestilentia à Rome: du tabu religieux à l'interprétation préscientifique', *Latomus* 39, 3–16.

Andreussi, M. (1996) 'Murus Servii Tullii; mura repubblicane', in E. M. Steinby (ed.), *Lexicon Topographicum Urbis Romae* 3: 319–24.

Andreussi, M. (1999) 'Pomerium', in E. M. Steinby (ed.), *Lexicon Topographicum Urbis Romae* 4, 96–105.

Applebaum, S. (1979) *Jews and Greeks in Ancient Cyrene*, Leiden.

Arce, J. (1990) *Funus Imperatorum: Los funerales de los emperadores romanos*, Madrid: Alianza.

Ariès, P. (1981) *The Hour of Our Death* (trans. of *L'Homme devant la Mort*, Paris, 1977), New York: Oxford University Press.

Avetta, L. (1985) *Roma – Via Imperiale*, Rome: edizioni di storia e letteratura.

Bacchielli, L. (1990) 'I luoghi della celebrazione politica e religiosa a Cirene nella poesia di Pindaro e Callimacho', in B. Gentili (ed.), *Cirene: Storia, mito, letteratura*, Urbino, 5–33.

Barrett, A. A. (1991) 'Claudius' British Victory Arch at Rome', *Britannia* 22, 1–20.

Barton, C. (1993) *Sorrows of the Ancient Romans: The Gladiator and the Monster*, Princeton: Princeton University Press.

Bauman, R. (1996) *Crime and Punishment in Ancient Rome*, London: Routledge.

Beard, M. (1998) 'Imaginary *horti*: or up the garden path', in M. Cima and E. La Rocca (eds), *Horti Romani: atti del convegno internazionale, Roma, 4–6 maggio 1995*, Rome: L'Erma di Bretschneider, 23–32.

Beard, M., North, J. and Price, S. (1998) *Religions of Rome*, 2 vols, Cambridge: Cambridge University Press.

Beavis, I. C. (1988) *Insects and Other Invertebrates in Classical Antiquity*, Exeter: University of Exeter Press.

Bell, W. G. (1924) *The Great Plague in London in 1665*, London: John Lane the Bodley Head.

Bernstein, A. (1993) *The Formation of Hell: Death and Retribution in the Ancient and Early Christian Worlds*, London: University College of London Press.

Bertrand, J.-M. (1988) 'Les Boucôloi ou le monde à l'envers', *Revue des Etudes Anciennes* 90, 139–49.

Bettini, M. (1986) *Antropologia e cultura romana. Parentela, tempo, immagini dell'anima*, Rome: Nuova Italia Scientifica.

Biraben, J.-N. (1975) *Les hommes et la peste en France et dans les pays européens et méditerranées*, 2 vols, Paris: École des Hautes Etudes en Sciences Sociales.
Bird, J., Claridge, A., Gilkes, O. and Neal, D. (1993) 'Porta Pia: Excavations and Survey in an Area of Suburban Rome, Part I', *Papers of the British School at Rome* 61, 51–114.
Birley, A. R. (1988) *The African Emperor: Septimius Severus*, London: Batsford.
Bisconti, F. (1999) 'Sepulcrum Aureli', in E. M. Steinby (ed.), *Lexicon Topographicum Urbis Romae* 4: 276–7.
Boatwright, M. T. (1984–5) 'Tacitus on Claudius and the Pomerium, *Annals* 12.23.2–24', *Classical Journal* 80, 36–43.
Boatwright, M. T. (1985) 'The "Ara Ditis – *Ustrinum* of Hadrian" in the Western Campus Martius and other Problematic Roman *ustrina*', *AJA* 89, 485–97.
Boatwright, M. T. (1986) 'The Pomerial Extensions of Augustus', *Historia* 35, 13–27.
Boatwright, M. T. (1987) *Hadrian and the City of Rome*, Princeton: Princeton University Press.
Bodel, J. (1994) 'Graveyards and Groves: A Study of the Lex Lucerina', *American Journal of Ancient History* 11, Cambridge, Mass.
Bodel, J. (1999) 'Death on Display: Looking at Roman Funerals', in B. Bergmann and C. Kondoleon (eds), *The Art of Ancient Spectacle*, Studies in the History of Art 56, Washington, DC: The National Gallery of Art, 258–81.
Boels, N. (1973) 'Le statut religieux de la Flaminica Dialis', *REL* 51, 77–100.
Boghurst, W. (1894) *Loimographia: An Account of the Great Plague of London in the Year 1665*, London.
Bollmann, B. (1997) 'La distribuzione delle scholae delle corporazioni a Roma', in *La Rome impériale: démographie et logistique = Collection de l'École Française de Rome* 230, 209–25.
Bollmann, B. (1998) *Römische Vereinshäuser*, Mainz: Philipp von Zabern.
Bömer, F. (1943) *Ahnenkult und Ahnenglaube im alten Rom*, Leipzig: Teubner.
Bonfante Warren, L. (1970) 'Roman Triumphs and Etruscan Kings: The Changing Face of the Triumph', *JRS* 60, 49–66.
Bonnefond-Coudry, M. (1989) *Le sénat de la république romaine*, Rome: École Française de Rome.
Bonniec, H. Le (1958) *Le culte de Cerès à Rome, des origines à la fin de la république*, Paris: Klincksieck.
Borca, F. (1994) ' "Udosis squalida terris": la palude come luogo del paradosso (Sil. 7. 277 s.)', *Lexis* 12, 151–6.
Borca, F. (1995a) 'Ai margini del "bel paesaggio": la percezione dell'ambiente palustre nella Roma antica', *Nuova Rivista Storica* 79, 245–60.
Borca, F. (1995b) 'Fondazione e fango: Romolo, la palude e le radici della cultura romana', *Aufidus* 26, 55–68.
Borca, F. (1995c) ' "Altae neu crede paludi": api e paludi in Verg. *Georg.* 4, 48 s.', *Sileno* 21, 161–5.
Borca, F. (1996a) ' "Adversus ipsam rerum naturam": Note on Tac. *Agr.* 33', *Britannia* 27, 337–40.
Borca, F. (1996b) ' "Stagna", "paludes" e presenza antropica. Il caso dell'alto Adriatico: un "unicum" nell'antichità classica?', *Quaderni di Storia* 44, 115–45.
Borca, F. (1996c) 'Uomini e paludi nella Gallia Narbonensis: insediamento, economia, mobilità', *Rivista di Studi Liguri* 62, 5–23.
Borca, F. (1996d) 'Due antiche etimologie di latino "palus, -udis" ', *Incontri linguistici* 19, 157–60.
Borca, F. (1996e) ' "Gnara vincentibus, iniqua nesciis palus": il soldato e l'acquitrino', *Geographia Antiqua* 5, 63–73.
Borca, F. (1997a) ' "Palus Omni Modo Vitanda": A Liminal Space in Ancient Roman Culture', *Classical Bulletin* 73, 3–12.

Borca, F. (1997b) 'Per uno studio del paesaggio germanico nella letteratura greco-latina', *Aufidus* 32, 41–59.

Borca, F. (1997c) ' "Vitabitur palustris vicinitas": un architetto alle prese con le paludi (riflessioni su alcuni passi vitruviani), *Quaderni Urbinati di Cultura Classica* 55, 49–58.

Borca, F. (1997d) 'Uomo e ambiente nella Gallia Cisalpina: il biotopo palustre nelle fonti letterarie antiche', *Bollettino storico-bibliografico Subalpino* 95, 5–26.

Borca, F. (1997e) ' "Garrula limosis rana coaxat aquis": la rana, il suo habitat e il gracidio', *Annali della Facoltà di Lettere e Filosofia dell'Università di Siena* 18, 151–76.

Borca, F. (1998) 'Il paesaggio nilotico nelle letterature greca e latina', *Materiali e discussioni per l'analisi dei testi classici* 41, 185–205.

Boyancé, P. (1952) 'Funus Acerbum', *REA* 54, 275–89.

Brown, S. (1992) 'Death as Decoration: Scenes from the Arena in Roman Domestic Mosaics', in A. Richlin (ed.), *Pornography and Representation in Greece and Rome*, Oxford: Oxford University Press: 180–211.

Brunt, P. A. (1973) 'Aspects of the Social Thought of Dio Chrysostom and of the Stoics', *PCPS* 19, 26–34.

Burkert, W. (1985) *Greek Religion* (trans. of *Griechische Religion der archäischen und klassichen Epoche*, Stuttgart, 1977), Oxford.

Buzzetti, C. (1993) 'Castra equitum singularium', in E. M. Steinby (ed.), *Lexicon Topographicum Urbis Romae* 1, 246–8.

Calame, C. (1986) 'Nature humaine et environnement: le racisme bien tempéré d'Hippocrate', in *Sciences et Racisme*, Lausanne: Publications de l'université Lausanne, 75–99.

Calame, C. (1990) 'Narrating the Foundation of a City: The Symbolic Birth of Cyrene', in L. Edmunds (ed.), *Approaches to Greek Myth*, Baltimore.

Campbell, J. B. (1984) *The Emperor and the Roman Army 31* BC–AD 235, *Oxford: Oxford University Press.*

Camporesi, P. (1989) *Bread of Dreams*, Oxford: Polity Press.

Cantarella, E. (1991) *I supplizi capitali in Grecia e a Roma*, Milan: Rizzoli.

Carandini, A. (1988) *Schiavi in Italia*, Rome: La Nuova Italia Scientifica.

Carandini, A. (1992) 'Le mura del Palatino, nuova fonte sulla Roma di età regia', *Bollettino di archeologia* 16–18, 1–18.

Carandini, A. (1997) *La nàscita di Roma*, Turin: Einaudi.

Carandini, A., Brocato, P., Carafa, P., Ricci, G. and Terrenato, N. (1992) 'Lo scavo delle mura palatine', *Bollettino di archeologia* 16–18, 111–38.

Carettoni, G., Colini, A. M., Cozza, L. and Gatti, G. (1960) *La pianta marmorea di Roma antica*, Rome: Danesi.

Carignani, A., Gabucci, A., Palazzo, P. and Spinola, G. (1990) 'Nuovi dati sulla topografia del Celio: le ricerche nell'area dell'ospedale militare', *Archeologia Laziale* 10 (1990), 72–80.

Carmichael, A. G. (1986) *Plague and the Poor in Renaissance Florence*, Cambridge: Cambridge University Press.

Carmichael, A. G. (1993) 'History of Public Health and Sanitation in the West before 1700', in K. Kiple (ed.), *The Cambridge World History of Human Disease*, Cambridge: Cambridge University Press.

Cassels, J. (1955) 'The Cemeteries of Cyrene', *Papers of the British School at Rome* 23 n.s. 10, 1–43.

Catalano, P. (1978) 'Aspetti spatiali del sistema giuridico religioso romano. Mundus, templum, urbs, ager, Latium, Italia', in H. Temporini and W. Haase (eds), *Aufstieg und Niedergang der römischen Welt*, Berlin: de Gruyter, 2.16.1: 442–553.

Chamoux, F. (1953) *Cyrene sous la monarchie des Battiades*, Paris.

Champlin, E. (1982) 'The Suburbium of Rome', *American Journal of Ancient History* 7, 97–117.
Champlin, E. (1991) *Final Judgements: Duty and Emotion in Roman Wills, 200 BC–AD 250*, Berkeley: University of California Press.
Cifani, G. (1997) 'Le mura arcaiche di Roma', in A. Carandini, *La nascita di Roma*, Turin: Einaudi, 623–7.
Cipolla, C. (1979) *I Pidocchi e il Granduca*, Bologna: Il Mulino.
Cipolla, C. (1981) *Fighting the Plague in Seventeenth-Century Italy*, Madison: University of Wisconsin Press.
Cipolla, C. (1992) *Miasmas and Disease*, New Haven and London: Yale University Press.
Clark, G. (1998) 'Bodies and Blood: Late Antique Debates on Martyrdom, Virginity and Resurrection', in D. Montserrat (ed.), *Changing Bodies, Changing Meanings: Studies on the Human Body in Antiquity*, London: Routledge, 99–115.
Coarelli, F. (1972) 'Il sepolcro degli Scipioni', *Dialoghi di Archeologia* 6, 36–106.
Coarelli, F. (1979) 'La Riscoperta del sepolcro degli Haterii. Una base con dedica a Silvano', in *Studies in Classical Art and Archaeology: A tribute to Peter Heinrich von Blanckenhagen*, Locust Valley, N.Y.: Augustin, 255–69.
Coarelli, F. (1985) *Il foro romano: periodo repubblicano e augusteo*, Rome: Quasar.
Coarelli, F. (1986) 'L'urbs e il suburbio', in A. Giardina (ed.), *Società romana e impero tardoantico*, Rome/Bari: Laterza, 2: 1–58.
Coarelli, F. (1988) 'Colonizzazione romana e viabilità', *Dialoghi di Archeologia*, 3rd series 6/2, 35–48.
Coarelli, F. (1992) 'Aedes Fortis Fortunae, Naumachia Augusti, Castra Ravennatium: la Via Campana Portuensis e alcuni edifici adiacenti nella pianta marmorea severiana', *Ostraka* 1, 39–54.
Coarelli, F. (1995a) *Guida Archeologica Laterza: Roma*, 2nd edn, Rome: Laterza.
Coarelli, F. (1995b) 'Fortuna Redux, ara', in E. M. Steinby (ed.), *Lexicon Topographicum Urbis Romae* 2, 275.
Coarelli, F. (1996a) 'Libitina, lucus', in E. M. Steinby (ed.), *Lexicon Topographicum Urbis Romae* 3.
Coarelli, F. (1996b) 'Murus Servii Tullii; Mura repubblicane: Porta Caelimontana', in E. M. Steinby (ed.), *Lexicon Topographicum Urbis Romae* 3, 324.
Coarelli, F. (1996c) 'Murus Servii Tullii; Mura repubblicane: Porta Capena', in E. M. Steinby (ed.), *Lexicon Topographicum Urbis Romae* 3, 325.
Coarelli, F. (1996d) 'Murus Servii Tullii; Mura repubblicane: Porta Esquilina', in E. M. Steinby (ed.), *Lexicon Topographicum Urbis Romae* 3, 327.
Coarelli, F. (1996e) 'Murus Servii Tullii; Mura repubblicane: Porta Flumentana', in E. M. Steinby (ed.), *Lexicon Topographicum Urbis Romae* 3, 327–8.
Coarelli, F. (1999a) 'Puticuli', in E. M. Steinby (ed.), *Lexicon Topographicum Urbis Romae* 4, 173–4.
Coarelli, F. (1999b) 'Senaculum', in E. M. Steinby (ed.), *Lexicon Topographicum Urbis Romae* 4, 264–5.
Coates-Stephens, R. (1998) 'The Walls and Aqueducts of Rome in the Early Middle Ages, AD 500–1000', *Journal of Roman Studies* 88, 166–78.
Cochrane, C. N. (1929) *Thucydides and the Science of History*, London.
Coleman, K. (1990) 'Fatal Charades: Roman Executions Staged as Mythological Enactments', *JRS* 80, 44–73.
Colini A. M. and Cozza, L. (1962) *Il ludus magnus*, Rome: Monte dei paschi di Siena.
Conlan, E. (1993) 'To the Potter's Field', *The New Yorker*, July 19, 42–54.
Connor, W. R. (1985) 'The Razing of the House in Greek society', *TAPA* 115, 79–102.
Corbin, A. (1982) *Le Miasme et la Jonquille*, Paris: Aubier Montaigne.
Corbin, A. (1986) *The Foul and the Fragrant*, Leamington Spa: Berg.

Corvisier, J. (1985) *Santé et société en Grèce ancienne*, Paris.

Counts, D. B. (1996) '*Regum externorum consuetudine*: The Nature and Function of Embalming in Rome' *CA* 15, 189–202.

Cozza, L. (1986) 'Mura Aureliane, I. Trastevere, il braccio settentrionale del Tevere a Porta Aurelia-S. Pancrazio', *Bullettino della Commissione Archeologica Comunale di Roma* 91, 103–30.

Crane, E. (1994) 'Beekeeping in the World of Ancient Rome', *Bee World* 75, 118–34.

Crane, E. and Graham, A. J. (1985) 'Bee Hives of the Ancient World. 1', *Bee World* 66, 34–9.

Crawford, M. H. (ed.) (1996) *Roman Statutes*, 2 vols (*BICS Supplement* 64), London: Institute of Classical Studies.

Crawfurd, R. (1914) *Plague and Pestilence in Literature and Art*, Oxford.

Cumont, F. (1937) *L'Égypte des astrologues*, Brussels: Fondation égyptologique reine Elisabeth.

Cuq, E. (1881) s.v. '*funus*', in C. Daremberg and E. Saglio (eds), *Dictionnaire des antiquités grecques et romaines d'après les textes et les monuments*, Paris.

D'Ambrosio, A. and De Caro, S. (1983) *Un impegno per Pompeii. Fotopiano e documentazione dell necropoli di Porta Nocera*, Rome: Touring Club Italiano.

David, J.-M. (1984) 'Du *comitium* à la roche Tarpéienne ... Sur certains rituels d'exécution capitale sous la république, les règnes d'Auguste et de Tibère', in *Du châtiment dans la cité: Supplices corporels et peine de mort dans le monde antique*, Paris: École Française de Rome, 131–76.

Debru, A. (ed.) (1997) *Galen on Pharmacology*, Leiden: Brill.

Delaine, J. (1995) 'The Supply of Building Materials to the City of Rome', in N. Christie (ed.), *Settlement and Economy in Italy 1500 BC–AD 1500*, Oxford: Oxbow, 555–62.

Della Corte, F. (1984) s.v. '*ape*', in *Enciclopedia Virgiliana* 1, Rome: Istituto della Enciclopedia Italiana, 213b–214a.

De Marchi, A. (1896) *Il culto privato di Roma antica*, vol. 1, Milan: U. Hoepli.

De Maria, S. (1988) *Gli archi onorari di Roma e dell'Italia romana*, Rome: l'Erma di Bretschneider.

Demont, P. (1983) 'Notes sur le récit de la pestilence athénienne chez Thucydide et sur ses rapports avec la médicine grecque de l'époque classique', in F. Lasserre and P. Mudry (eds), *Formes de pensée dans la collection hippocratique*, Geneva, 341–53.

Dent, J. (1985) 'Burial Practices in Cyrenaica', in G. Barker, J. Lloyd and J. Reynold, (eds), *Cyrenaica in Antiquity*, Society for Libyan Studies Occasional Papers 1, BAR International Series 236, 327–36.

Derda, T. (1991) 'Necropolis Workers in Graeco-Roman Egypt in the Light of the Greek Papyri', *JJP* 21, 13–36.

De Ruyt, C. (1983) *Macellum: marché alimentaire des romains*, = *Publications d'histoire de l'art et d'archéologie de l'Université catholique de Louvain* 35.

Deschamps, L. (1995) 'Rites funéraires de la Rome républicaine', in F. Hinard (ed.), *La mort au quotidien dans le monde Romain*, Paris: De Boccard, 171–80.

Desideri, P. (1995) 'Il trattamento del corpo dei suicidi', in F. Hinard (ed.), *La mort au quotidien dans le monde Romain*, Paris: De Boccard, 189–204.

De Visscher, F. (1963) *Le droit des tombeaux romains*, Milan: Giuffrè.

Dodds, E. R. (1959) *Plato: Gorgias*, Oxford: Clarendon Press.

D'Onofrio, C. (1967) *Gli obelischi di Roma*, 2nd edn, Rome: Bulzoni.

Dougherty, C. (1993) *The Poetics of Colonization: From City to Text in Archaic Greece*, Oxford.

Dougherty, C. (1994) 'Archaic Greek Foundation Poetry: Questions of Genre and Occasion', *JHS* 114, 35–46.

Douglas, M. (1968) 'Pollution', in D. L. Sills (ed.), *International Encyclopedia of the Social Sciences*, New York: Crowell, Collier and Macmillan.

Dover, K. (1975) 'The Freedom of the Intellectual in Greek Society', *Talanta* 7.

Ducos, M. (1995) 'Le tombeau, *locus religiosus*', in F. Hinard (ed.), *La mort au quotidien dans le monde Romain*, Paris: De Boccard, 135–44.

Ducrey, P. (1995) 'La muraille est-elle un élément constitutif d'une cité?', in *Sources for the Ancient Greek City-State, Symposium August 24–27 1994, Acts of the Copenhagen Polis Centre*, vol. 2, Copenhagen, 245–56.

Dumont, J.-C. (1995) 'L'enlèvement du cadavre', in F. Hinard (ed.), *La mort au quotidien dans le monde Romain*, Paris: De Boccard, 181–7.

Durry, M. (1968) *Les cohortes prétoriennes*, 2nd edn, Paris: E. de Boccard.

Eck, W. (1988) 'Aussagefähigkeit epigraphischer Statistik und die Bestattung von Sklaven im kaiserzeitlichen Rom', in P. Kneissl and V. Losemann (eds), *Alte Geschichte und Wissenschaftsgeschichte. Festschrift für Karl Christ*, Darmstadt: Wissenschaftliche Buchgesellschaft: 30–9.

Eck, W. (1997) 'Cum dignitate otium: Senatorial Domus in Imperial Rome', *Scripta Classica Israelitica* 19, 162–90.

Edelstein, L. (1967) 'The History of Anatomy in Antiquity', in C. Temkin and O. Temkin (eds), *Ancient Medicine: Selected Papers of Ludwig Edelstein*, Baltimore: Johns Hopkins Press, 247–301.

Edwards, C. (1997) 'Unspeakable Professions: Public Performance and Prostitution in Ancient Roma', in J. P. Hallett and M. B. Skinner (eds), *Roman Sexualities*, Princeton: Princeton University Press, 66–95.

Ernout, A. and Meillet, A. (1959) *Dictionnaire étymologique de la langue latine*, 4th edn, Paris: Librairie C. Klincksieck.

Favro, D. (1996) *The Urban Image of Augustan Rome*, Cambridge: Cambridge University Press.

Fedeli, P. (1990) *La natura violata. Ecologia e mondo romano*, Palermo: Sellerio.

Felton, D. (1999) *Haunted Greece and Rome: Ghost Stories from Classical Antiquity*, Austin: University of Texas Press.

Floriani Squarciapino, M. (1956) *Scavi di Ostia III. Le necropoli*, Rome: Libreria dello Stato.

Flower, H. I. (1996) *Ancestor Masks and Aristocratic Power in Roman Culture*, Oxford: Clarendon Press.

Fontana, F. (1999) 'Sepulcrum: Valerii', in E. M. Steinby (ed.), *Lexicon Topographicum Urbis Romae* 4, 301.

Forcella, E. (1984) 'Il cimitero del Verano', in *Architettura e urbanistica. Uso e trasformazione della città storica* (Roma Capitale 1870–1911, vol. 7), Rome: Marsilio, 276–91.

Frank, J. P. (1780) *System einer vollständigen medizinischen Polizey*, Mannheim: C. F. Schwan.

Frank, J. P. (1976) *A System of Complete Medical Police*, Baltimore: Johns Hopkins University Press.

Frazer, J. (1934–6) *The Fear of the Dead in Primitive Religion*, vols 1–3, London: Macmillan.

Freyburger, G. (1995) 'Libitine et les funérailles', in F. Hinard (ed.), *La mort au quotidien dans le monde Romain*, Paris: De Boccard, 213–22.

Frézouls, E. (1987) 'Rome ville ouverte. Réflexions sur les problèmes de l'expansion urbaine d'Auguste à Aurélien', in *L'Urbs: espace urbain et histoire*, = *Collection de l'École Française de Rome* 98, 373–92.

Gabba, E. (1983) 'La rifondazione di Salapia', *Athenaeum* 61, 514–16.

Gager, J. (1992) *Curse Tablets and Binding Spells from the Ancient World*, Oxford: Oxford University Press.

Gardner, J. (1993) *Being a Roman Citizen*, London: Routledge.

Gardner, J. and Wiedemann, T. (1991) *The Roman Household: A Sourcebook*, London: Routledge.

Garland, R. (1985) *The Greek Way of Death*, London: Duckworth.

Garland, R. (1989) 'The Well-Ordered Corpse: An Investigation into the Motives behind Greek Funerary Legislation', *BICS* 36, 1–15.

Gatrell, V. (1994) *The Hanging Tree: Execution and the English People 1770–1868*, Oxford: Oxford University Press.

Giannini, P. (1990) 'Cirene nella posia greca: tra mito e storia', in B. Gentili (ed.), *Cirene: Storia, mito, letteratura*, Urbino, 51–95.

Giardina, A. (1997) *L'Italia romana: storia di un'identità incompiuta*, Rome/Bari: Laterza.
Gilkes, O. J., Passigli, S. and Schinke, R. (1994) 'Porta Pia: Excavation and Survey in an Area of Suburban Rome, Part II', *Papers of the British School at Rome* 62, 101–38.
Ginouvès, R., Guimier-Sorbets, A.-M., Jouanna, J. and Villard, L. (1994) *L'Eau, la Santé et la Maladie dans le Monde grec*, Paris: Ecole Française d'Athènes.
Gittings, C. (1984) *Death, Burial, and the Individual in Early Modern England*, London: Croom Helm.
Giuliano, A. (1968) 'Documenti per servire allo studio del monumento degli "Haterii"', *Memorie della Accademia Nazionale dei Lincei* (Series 8) 13, 449–82.
Gomme, A. (1956) *A Historical Commentary on Thucydides*, vol. 2, Oxford: Clarendon Press.
Goodchild, R. (1952) 'Mapping Roman Libya', *Geographical Journal* 118, 142–52.
Goodchild, R. (1953) 'The Roman and Byzantine *Limes* in Cyrenaica', *JRS* 43, 65–76.
Goodchild, R. (1971) *Kyrene und Apollonia*, Zurich.
Graham, A. J. (1964) *Colony and Mother City in Ancient Greece*, Manchester.
Grainger, R. (1998) *The Social Symbolism of Grief and Mourning*, London: Jessica Kingsley.
Grandazzi, A. (1991) 'Les mots et les choses: la composition du De Verborum Significatu de Verrius Flaccus', *REL* 69, 101–23.
Granger, F. (1962) *Vitruvius, On Architecture*, 1, London and Cambridge, Mass.: Harvard University Press.
Griffin, M. T. (1962) '*De brevitate vitae*', *JRS* 52, 104–13.
Grmek, M. D. (1991) *Diseases in the Ancient Greek World*, trans. M. Muellner and L. Muellner, Baltimore.
Gwyn Morgan, M. (1974) 'Priests and Physical Fitness', *CQ* 24, 137–41.
Häuber, C. (1990) 'Zur Topographie der Horti Maecenatis und der Horti Lamiani auf dem Esquilin in Rom', *Kölner Jahrbuch für Vor- und Frühgeschichte* 23, 11–107.
Häuber, C. (1996) 'Horti Maecenatis', in E. M. Steinby (ed.), *Lexicon Topographicum Urbis Romae* 3, 70–4.
Hesberg, H. von (1989) 'Vitruv und die Stadtplanung in spätrepublikanischer und augustischer Zeit', in H. Geertman and J. J. De Jong (eds), *Munus non ingratum: Proceedings of the International Symposium on Vitruvius' De Architectura and the Hellenistic and Republican Architecture, Leiden 20–23 January 1987*, Leiden: Brill, 134–40.
Hesberg, H. von (1994) *Monumenta: i sepolcri romani e la loro architettura*, Milan: Longanesi.
Hesberg, V. von (1992) *Römische Grabbauten*, Darmstadt: Wissenschaftliche Buchgesellschaft.
Heskell, J. (1994) 'Cicero as Evidence for Attitudes to Dress in the Late Republic', in J. Sebesta and L. Bonfante (eds), *The World of Roman Costume*, Madison: University of Wisconsin Press.
Hinard, F. (1976) 'Remarques sur les *praecones* et le *praeconium* dans la Rome de la fin de la République', *Latomus* 35, 730–46.
Hinard, F. (1987) 'Spectacle des exécutions et espace urbain', in *L'Urbs. Espace urbain et histoire (Ier siècle av. J.-C. – IIIe siècle ap. J.-C)*, Rome: École Francaise de Rome: 111–25.
Hinard, F. (1995) 'La "Loi de Pouzzoles" et les pompes funèbres', in F. Hinard (ed.), *La mort au quotidien dans le monde Romain*, Paris: De Boccard, 205–12.
Holleman, A. W. J. (1973) 'An Enigmatic Function of the Flamen Dialis (Ovid *Fast.* 2.282) and the Augustan Reform', *Numen* 20, 222–8.
Hooper, W. D. (1934) *Marcus Porcius Cato, On Agriculture. Marcus Terentius Varro, On Agriculture*, London and Cambridge, Mass.: Harvard University Press.
Hope, V. (1997) 'A Roof over the Dead: Communal Tombs and Family Structure', in R. Laurence and A. Wallace-Hadrill (eds), *Domestic Space in the Roman World: Pompeii and Beyond*, *JRA* Supplementary Series 22, 69–88.
Hope, V. (1998) 'Negotiating Identity and Status: The Gladiators of Roman Nîmes', in J. Berry and R. Laurence (eds), *Cultural Identity in the Roman Empire*, London: Routledge, 179–95.

Hope, V. (forthcoming) 'Fighting for Identity: The Funerary Commemoration of Italian Gladiators', in A. Cooley (ed.), *The Epigraphic Landscape of Roman Italy*, *BICS* Supplement.
Hopkins, K. (1978) *Conquerors and Slaves*, Cambridge: Cambridge University Press.
Hopkins, K. (1983) *Death and Renewal*, Sociological Studies in Roman History, 2, Cambridge: Cambridge University Press.
Hornblower, S. (1987) *Thucydides*, London: Duckworth.
Hornblower, S. (1991) *A Commentary on Thucydides I: Books I–III*, Oxford: Clarendon Press.
Horsfall, N. (1983) 'Some Problems in the "Laudatio Turiae"', *BICS* 30, 85–98.
How, W. W. and Wells, J. (1912) *A Commentary on Herodotus*, Oxford: Clarendon Press.
Howell, P. (1980) *A Commentary on Book One of the Epigrams of Martial*, London: Athlone Press.
Hughes, J. D. (1994) *Pan's Travail: Environmental Problems of the Ancient Greeks and Romans*, Baltimore and London: The Johns Hopkins University Press.
Huntington, R. and Metcalf, P. (1979) *Celebrations of Death*, Cambridge: Cambridge University Press.
Hyslop, G. C. (1945) *Cyrene and Ancient Cyrenaica*, Tripoli.
Jackson, R. (1988) *Doctors and Diseases in the Roman Empire*, London: British Museum.
Jenkins, G. K. (1974) 'Some Ancient Coins of Libya', *Libyan Studies* 5, 29–34.
Johnson, E. L. (1988) 'Funeral Laments of Hakka Women', in J. L. Watson and E. S. Rawski (eds), *Death Ritual in Late Imperial and Modern China*, California: California University Press: 135–63.
Jones, C. P. (1987) '*Stigma*: Tattooing and Branding in Graeco-Roman Antiquity', *JRS* 77, 139–55.
Jones, H. L. (1923; 1932) *The Geography of Strabo*, II–VIII, London and New York: Harvard University Press.
Jones, W. H. S. (1923) *Hippocrates*, I, London and New York: Harvard University Press.
Josi, E. (1950) 'Cimiteri Cristiani Antichi', *Enciclopedia Cattolica* 3, 1617–37.
Jouanna, J. (1978) 'Le médecin modèle du législateur dans les *Lois* de Platon', *Ktema* 3, 77–91.
Jouanna, J. (1980) 'Politique et médecine. La problématique du changement dans *le Régime des maladies aiguës* et chez Thucydide (livre VI)', in M. D. Grmek (ed.), *Hippocratica*, Paris: CNRS, 299–318.
Jouanna, J. (1996) *Hippocrate, Airs, Eaux, Lieux*, Paris: Les Belles Lettres.
Kajanto, I. (1965) *The Latin Cognomina*, Helsinki: Societas Scientiarum Fennica (Commentationes Humanarum Literarum).
Kallet, L. (1999) 'The Diseased Body Politic, Athenian Public Finance, and the Massacre at Mykalessos (Thucydides 7.27–29)', *AJP* 120, 223–44.
Kierdorf, W. (1980) *Laudatio Funebris. Interpretationen und Untersuchungen zur Entwicklung der römischen Leichenrede*, Meisenheim: Anton Hein (Beitrage zur klassischen Philologie 106).
Kiple, K. F. (ed.) (1993) *The Cambridge World History of Human Disease*, Cambridge: Cambridge University Press.
Knobloch, J. (1991) 'Überlegungen zur Deutung von lat. *vespillo* "νεκροθάπτης"-*sandapilarius*"', *RhM* 134, 403–4.
Kockel, V. (1983) *Die Grabbauten vor dem Herkulaner Tor in Pompeji*, Mainz: Philipp von Zabern.
Kollesch, J. and Nickel, D. (eds) (1993) *Galen und das hellenistische Erbe*, Stuttgart: Franz Steiner Verlag.
Kurtz, D. and Boardman, J. (1971) *Greek Burial Customs*, London: Thames and Hudson.
Kyle, D. G. (1998) *Spectacles of Death in Ancient Rome*, London and New York: Routledge.
Labrousse, M. (1937) 'Le pomerium de la Rome impériale', *Mél. Arch. Hist.* 54, 165–99.
Lanciani, R. (1874) 'Puticoli', *BCAR* 2, 42–53.
Lanciani, R. (1875) 'Le antichissime sepolture Esquiline', *BCAR* 3, 41–56.
Lanciani, R. (1888) *Ancient Rome in the Light of Recent Discoveries*, Urbana: University of Illinois.

Lanciani, R. (1890) *Ancient Rome in the Light of Recent Discoveries*, Boston and New York: Houghton, Mifflin and Co.

Langholf, V. (1990) *Medical Theories in Hippocrates: Early Texts and the 'Epidemics'*, Berlin.

Laqueur, T. (1983) 'Bodies, Death, and Pauper Funerals', *Representations* 1, 109–31.

Laronde, A. (1987) *Cyrene et la Libye Hellenistique. LIBYKAI HISTOIAI. De l'epoque republicaine au principat d'Auguste*, Paris.

Laurence, R. (1993) 'Emperors, Nature and the City: Rome's Ritual Landscape', *Accordia Research Papers* 4, 79–88.

Lavagne, H. (1987) 'Le tombeau, mémoire du mort', in F. Hinard (ed.), *La mort, les morts et l'au delà dans le monde romain,* Caen: Université de Caen, 159–65.

Lega, C. (1999) 'Septem Caesares', in E. M. Steinby (ed.), *Lexicon Topographicum Urbis Romae* 4, 266.

Le Gall, J. (1991) 'La muraille servienne sous le Haut-Empire', in F. Hinard and M. Royo (eds), *Rome: l'espace urbain et ses représentations*, Paris: Presses de l'Université de Paris-Sorbonne, 55–64.

Leven, K. H. (1993) 'Miasma und Metadosis – antike Vorstellungen von Ansteckung', *Medizin, Gesellschaft und Geschichte* 11, 44–73.

Levick, B. M. (1983) 'The *Senatus Consultum* from Larinum', *JRS* 73, 97–115.

Levick, B. M. (1990) *Claudius*, London: Batsford.

Lichtenthaeler, C. (1979) 'οὔτε γὰρ ἰατροὶ ἤρκουν τὸ πρῶτον θεραπεύοντες ἀγνοίᾳ' *Hermes* 107/3, 270–86.

Lindsay, H. M. (1996) 'The Romans and Ancestor Worship', in M. Dillon (ed.), *Religion in the Ancient World: New Themes and Approaches*, Amsterdam: Hakkert, 271–85.

Lindsay, H. M. (1998) 'Eating with the Dead: The Roman Funerary Banquet', in I. Nielsen and H. S. Nielsen (eds), *Meals in a Social Context*, Aarhus Studies in Mediterranean Antiquity 1, Aarhus: Aarhus University Press, 67–80.

Linebaugh, P. (1975) 'The Tyburn Riot against the Surgeons', in D. Hay (ed.), *Albion's Fatal Tree: Crime and Society in Eighteenth-Century England*, London: Penguin, 65–117.

Lintott, A. (1999) *The Constitution of the Roman Republic*, Oxford, Oxford University Press.

Lissi Caronna, E. (1993a) 'Castra peregrina', in E. M. Steinby (ed.), *Lexicon Topographicum Urbis Romae* 1, 249–51.

Lissi Caronna, E. (1993b) 'Castra praetoria', in E. M. Steinby (ed.), *Lexicon Topographicum Urbis Romae* 1, 251–4.

Loane, H. J. (1938) *Industry and Commerce of the City of Rome (50 BC–200 AD)*, Baltimore: Johns Hopkins University Press.

Lo Cascio, E. (1975–6) '*Praeconium* e *dissignatio* nella *Tabula Heracleensis*', *Helikon* 15–16, 351–71.

Lo Cascio, E. (1994) 'The Size of the Roman Population: Beloch and the Meaning of the Augustan Census Figures', *JRS* 84, 23–40.

Longmate, N. (1966) *King Cholera*, London.

Longo, O. (1975) 'La polis, la mura, le navi (Tucidide 7.77.7)', *Quaderni di Storia* 1, 87–113.

Longrigg, J. (1980) 'The Great Plague of Athens', *History of Science* 18.

Longrigg, J. (1992) 'Epidemic, Ideas and Classical Athenian Society', in T. Ranger and P. Slack (eds), *Epidemics and Ideas: Essays on the Historical Perception of Pestilence*, Cambridge, 21–44.

Longrigg, J. (1993) *Greek Rational Medicine*, London: Routledge.

Longrigg, J. (1994) 'Empedocles and the Plague of Selinus: A Cock and Bull Story?', in *Tria Lustra: A Festschrift in Honour of John Pinsent*, Liverpool.

López Férez, J. A. (1992) 'La medicine meteorologique dans la collection hippocratique', in A. Thivel (ed.), *Actes du IIe colloque sur la pensée antique, organisé par le C.R.H.I.*, Paris, 207–22.

Luck, G. (1985) *Arcana Mundi: Magic and the Occult in the Greek and Roman Worlds*, Baltimore and London: Johns Hopkins University Press.

Lugli, G. (1952) *Fontes ad topographiam veteris urbis Romae pertinentes*, Rome: Università di Roma, Istituto di topografia antica.
Macdonald, M. and Murphy, T. (1990) *Sleepless Souls: Suicide in Early Modern England*, Oxford: Clarendon Press.
McKinley, J. I. (1989) 'Cremations: Expectations, Methodologies, and Realities', in C. A. Roberts, F. Lee and J. Birtliff (eds), *Burial Archaeology: Current Research, Methods, and Development*, BAR British Series 211, 65–76.
McManners, J. (1981) *Death and the Enlightenment: Changing Attitudes to Death among Christians and Unbelievers in Eighteenth-Century France*, Oxford: Oxford University Press.
McQueen, E. I. (1986) *Demosthenes: Olynthiacs*, Bristol: Bristol Classical Press.
Malinowski, B. (1925) 'Magic, Science and Religion', in J. Needham (ed.), *Science, Religion and Reality*, London: Macmillan.
Malinowski, B. (1954) *Magic, Science and Religion*, repr. New York: Doubleday.
Marx, K. F. H. (1824) *Origines Contagii*, Karlsruhe: D. R. Marx.
Marx, K. F. H. (1926) *Additamenta ad Origines Contagii,* Karlsruhe: D. R. Marx.
Mingazzini, P. (1966) *L'insula di Giasone Magno a Cirene*, Rome.
Missiou, A. (1992) *The Subversive Oratory of Andokides*, Cambridge.
Moggi, M. (1983) 'L'Elemento Indigeno nella Tradizione Letteraria sulle *ktiseis*', in *Modes de contact et processus de transformation dans les societes anciennes*, 979–1004.
Mols, R. (1954–6) *Introduction à la démographie historique des villes d'Europe du XIVe au XVIIIe siècle*, 3 vols, Louvain: Éditions J. Duculot, S. A., Gembloux.
Mommsen, Th. (1887–8) *Römisches Staatsrecht*, 3 vols: I^3, II^3, III.1 (1887), III.2 (1888), Leipzig.
Mommsen, Th. (1895) 'Zum römischen Grabrecht', *ZRG* 16, 203–20 [= *Ges. Schriften* 3.198–214].
Mommsen, Th. (1899) *Römisches Strafrecht*, Leipzig.
Montserrat, D. (1997) 'Death and Funerals in the Roman Fayum', in M. L. Bierbrier (ed.), *Portraits and Masks: Burial Customs in Roman Egypt*, London: British Museum, 33–44.
Montserrat, D. (ed.) (1998) *Changing Bodies, Changing Meanings: Studies on the Human Body in Antiquity*, London: Routledge.
Morel, J. P. (1987) 'La topographie de l'artisanat et du commerce dans la Rome antique', in *L'urbs: espace urbain et histoire = Collection de l'École Française de Rome* 98, 127–55.
Morley, N. (1996) *Metropolis and Hinterland: The City of Rome and the Italian Economy, 200 BC–AD 200*, Cambridge: Cambridge University Press.
Morris, I. (1992) *Death-Ritual and Social Structure in Classical Antiquity*, Cambridge: Cambridge University Press.
Morris, R. J. (1976) *Cholera 1832: The Social Response to an Epidemic*, London: Croom Helm.
Müller, K. E. (1972) *Geschichte der antiken Ethnographie und ethnologischen Theoriebildung von den Anfängen bis auf die byzantinischen Historiographen*, 1, Wiesbaden: Franz Steiner.
Mustakallio, K. (1994) *Death and Disgrace: Capital Penalties with Post Mortem Sanctions in Early Roman Historiography*, Annales Academiae Scientiarum Fennicae Dissertationes Humanarum Litterarum 72, Helsinki.
Needham, R. (1967) 'Percussion and Transition', *Man* n.s. 2, 606–14.
Néraudau, J.-P. (1984) *Etre Enfant à Rome*, Paris: Les Belles Lettres.
Nestle, W. (1927) 'Die Fabel des Menenius Agrippa', *Klio* 21, 350–60.
Nicaise, F. (1980) *La Grande Chirurgie*, Paris.
Nicolet, C. (1966) *L'ordre équestre à l'époque républicaine*, 2 vols, Paris.
Nicolet, C. (1991) *Space, Geography and Politics in the Early Roman Empire*, Ann Arbor: University of Michigan Press.
Nippel, W. (1995) *Public Order in Ancient Rome*, Cambridge: Cambridge University Press.
Noy. D. (forthcoming) ' "Half-burnt on an Emergency Pyre": Roman Cremations which Went Wrong'.

Nutton, V. (1981) 'The Seeds of Disease: An Explanation of Contagion and Infection from the Greeks to the Renaissance', *Medical History* 27, 1–34.

Nutton, V. (1992) 'Healers in the Medical Market Place', in A. G. Wear, (ed.), *Medicine in Society*, Cambridge: Cambridge University Press.

Nutton, V. (1993) 'Galen and Egypt', in J. Kollesch and D. Nickel (eds), *Galen und das hellenistische Erbe*, Stuttgart: Franz Steiner Verlag.

Nutton, V. (1995) 'Galen *ad multos annos*', *Dynamis* 15, 25–39.

Nutton, V. (1997) 'Galen on Theriac: Problems of Authenticity', in A. Debru (ed.) (1997) *Galen on Pharmacology,* Leiden: Brill.

Nutton, V. (1999) 'Did the Greeks have a Word for it? Contagion and Contagion Theory in Classical Antiquity', in L. I. Conrad (ed.), *Contagion and Infection in Pre-modern Societies*, London: Routledge.

Oriolo, F. (1999) 'Sepulcrum: Fabricii', in E. M. Steinby (ed.), *Lexicon Topographicum Urbis Romae* 4: 288–9.

Ostwald, M. (1969) *Nomos and the Beginnings of the Athenian Democracy*, Oxford: Clarendon Press.

Pailler, J.-M and Sablayrolles, R. (1994) 'Damnatio memoriae: une vraie perpetuité?', *Pallas* 40, 11–55.

Palmer, R. E. A. (1980) 'Customs on Market Goods Imported into the City of Rome', in J. H. D'Arms and E. C. Kopff (eds), *The Seaborne Commerce of Ancient Rome: Studies in Archaeology and History*, Rome: American Academy: 217–34.

Palmer, R. E. A. (1981) 'The Topography and Social History of Rome's Trastevere (Southern Sector)', *Proceedings of the American Philosophical Society* 125, 368–97.

Palmer, R. J. (1978) *The Control of Plague in Venice and Northern Italy*, Ph.D. Diss., University of Kent at Canterbury.

Palombi, D. (1993a) 'Arcus Traiani', in E. M. Steinby (ed.), *Lexicon Topographicum Urbis Romae* 1, 112.

Palombi, D. (1993b) 'Arcus Divi Veri', in E. M. Steinby (ed.), *Lexicon Topographicum Urbis Romae* 1, 112.

Palombi, D. (1996) 'Honos et Virtus, Aedes', in E. M. Steinby (ed.), *Lexicon Topographicum Urbis Romae* 3, 31–3.

Panciera, S. (1994) *Das Mausoleum des Augustus. Der Bau und seine Inschriften*, Munich.

Parisi Presicce, C. (1994) 'La dea con il silphio e l'iconographia di Panakeia a Cirene', in J. Reynolds (ed.), *Cyrenaican Archaeology: An International Colloquium*, *Libyan Studies* 25, 85–100.

Parker, R. (1983) *Miasma: Pollution and Purification in Early Greek Religion*, Oxford: Clarendon Press.

Parkin, T. G. (1992) *Demography and Roman Society*, Baltimore: Johns Hopkins University Press.

Parry, A. (1969) 'The Language of Thucydides' Description of the Plague', *BICS* 16, 106–18 (= in P. H. J. Lloyd-Jones (ed.), *The Language of Achilles and Other Papers*, Oxford: Clarendon Press, 1989, 156–76).

Parry, J. (1980) 'Ghosts, Greed and Sin: The Occupational Identity of the Benares Funeral Priests', *Man* n.s. 15, 88–111.

Patterson, J. R. (1992) 'Patronage, *collegia* and Burial in Imperial Rome', in S. Bassett (ed.), *Death in Towns: Urban Responses to the Dying and the Dead, 100–1600*, Leicester: Leicester University Press, 15–27.

Patterson, J. R. (2000) *Political Life in the City of Rome*, Bristol: Bristol Classical Press.

Patterson, J. R. (forthcoming a) 'Via Appia', in E. M. Steinby (ed.), *Lexicon Topographicum Urbis Romae* 5.

Patterson, J. R. (forthcoming b) 'Via Lata', in E. M. Steinby (ed.), *Lexicon Topographicum Urbis Romae* 5.

Perdrizet, P. (1934) 'La mort qui sentait bien', in *Mélanges Bidez*, Brussels, 719–27.

Petracca, L. and Vigna, L. M. (1985) 'Le fornaci di Roma e suburbio', in *Misurare la terra: centuriazione e coloni nel mondo romano. Città, agricoltura, commercio: materiali da Roma e dal suburbio*, Modena: Panini, 131–7.

Phillips, J. H. (1982) 'On Varro's *animalia quaedam minuta* and Etiology of Disease', *Transl. and Stud. of the College of Physicians of Philadelphia* 4, 12–25.

Pietrangeli, C. (1940) 'Via Prenestina, "il Torrione" ', *BCAR* 68, 239–43.

Pinault, J. R. (1992) *Hippocratic Lives and Legends*, Leiden, New York and Köln.

Pisani Sartorio, G. (1993) 'Arcus Drusi (Via Appia)', in E. M. Steinby (ed.), *Lexicon Topographicum Urbis Romae* 1, 93.

Pisani Sartorio, G. (1996a) 'Macellum', in E. M. Steinby (ed.), *Lexicon Topographicum Urbis Romae* 3, 201–3.

Pisani Sartorio, G. (1996b) 'Macellum Liviae', in E. M. Steinby (ed.), *Lexicon Topographicum Urbis Romae* 3, 203–4.

Pisani Sartorio, G. (1996c) 'Macellum Magnum', in E. M. Steinby (ed.), *Lexicon Topographicum Urbis Romae* 3, 204–6.

Pisani Sartorio, G. (1996d) 'Muri Aureliani', in E. M. Steinby (ed.), *Lexicon Topographicum Urbis Romae* 3, 290–9.

Pisani Sartorio, G. (1996e) 'Mutatorium Caesaris', in E. M. Steinby (ed.), *Lexicon Topographicum Urbis Romae* 3, 335.

Pisani Sartorio, G. (1999) 'Septizodium', in E. M. Steinby (ed.), *Lexicon Topographicum Urbis Romae* 4, 269–72.

Pisani Sartorio, G. and Quilici Gigli, S. (1987–8) 'A proposito della Tomba dei Corneli', *Bullettino della commissione archeologica comunale di Roma* 92, 247–64.

Plass, P. (1995) *The Game of Death in Ancient Rome: Arena Sport and Political Suicide*, Wisconsin: University of Wisconsin Press.

Pleket, H. W. (1995) 'The Social Status of Physicians in the Roman World', in P. J. van der Eijk, H. F. J. Horstmanshoff and P. H. Schrijvers (eds), *Ancient Medicine in its Socio-Cultural Context*, Amsterdam: Rodopi.

Poole, J. C. F. and Holladay, A. J. (1979) 'Thucydides and the Plague of Athens', *CQ* 29, 282–300.

Pötscher, W. (1968) 'Flamen Dialis', *Mnemosyne* 21, 215–39.

Price, S. (1987) 'From Noble Funerals to Divine Cult: The Consecration of the Roman Emperors', in D. Cannadine and S. Price (eds), *Rituals of Royalty: Power and Ceremonial in Traditional Societies*, Cambridge: Cambridge University Press, 56–105.

Pronti, A. (1993) 'Coraria Septimiana', in E. M. Steinby (ed.), *Lexicon Topographicum Urbis Romae* 1, 322–3.

Purcell, N. (1987) 'Tomb and Suburb', in H. von Hesberg and P. Zanker (eds), *Römische Gräberstraßen. Status, Standard, Selbstdarstellungen*, Munich: Bayerische Akademie der Wissenschaften, 25–41.

Purcell, N. (1995) 'Forum Romanum (The Republican Period)', in E. M. Steinby (ed.), *Lexicon Topographicum Urbis Romae* 2, 333–5.

Radke, G. (1973) 'Viae publicae romanae', in *Paulys Realencyclopädie der classischen Altertumswissenschaft*, Supplementband 13, Munich: Alfred Druckmüller, 1494–1534.

Rechenauer, G. (1991) *Thucydides und die hippokratische Medizin*, Hildesheim and New York.

Richardson. L. (1992) *A New Topographical Dictionary of Ancient Rome*, Baltimore and London: Johns Hopkins University Press.

Richardson, R. (1988) *Death, Dissection and the Destitute*, London: Penguin.

Richmond, I. A. (1930) *The City Wall of Imperial Rome*, Oxford: Oxford University Press.

Robinson, E. S. G. (1927) *A Catalogue of the Greek Coins in the British Museum*, London.

Robinson, O. (1975) 'The Roman Law on Burials and Burial Grounds', *The Irish Jurist* 10, 175–186.

Robinson, O. F. (1992) *Ancient Rome: City Planning and Administration*, London and New York: Routledge.

de Romilly, J. (1976) 'Alcibiade et le mélange entre jeunes et vieux: politique et médecine', *WS* n.s. 10, 93–105.

Rodriguez Almeida, E. (1981) *Forma urbis marmorea: aggiornamento generale 1980*, Rome: Quasar.

Rodriguez Almeida, E. (1993a) 'Arcus Claudii (a. 43 d.C.)', in E. M. Steinby (ed.), *Lexicon Topographicum Urbis Romae* 1, 85–6.

Rodriguez Almeida, E. (1993b) 'Area Carruces', in E. M. Steinby (ed.), *Lexicon Topographicum Urbis Romae* 1, 118.

Rodriguez Almeida, E. (1993c) 'Area Radicaria', in E. M. Steinby (ed.), *Lexicon Topographicum Urbis Romae* 1, 119–20.

Rodriguez Almeida, E. (1993d) 'Camenae', in E. M. Steinby (ed.), *Lexicon Topographicum Urbis Romae* 1, 216.

Rodriguez Almeida, E. (1993e) 'Cellae Vinariae Nova et Arruntiana', in E. M. Steinby (ed.), *Lexicon Topographicum Urbis Romae* 1, 259.

Rose, H. J. (1923) 'Nocturnal Funerals in Rome', *CQ* 17, 191–4.

Rosen, G. (1993) *A History of Public Health*, enlarged edn, Baltimore: Johns Hopkins University Press.

Rush, A. C. (1941) *Death and Burial in Christian Antiquity*, diss., Catholic University of America, Washington D.C.

Rushton, G. (1915) 'Funeral Lights in Roman Sepulchral Monuments', *JRS* 5, 149–64.

Russo, J., Fernández-Galiano, M. and Heubeck, A. (1992) *A Commentary on Homer's Odyssey*, vol. 3, Oxford.

Rykwert, J. (1976) *The Idea of a Town: The Anthropology of Urban Form in Rome, Italy and the Ancient World*, Princeton: Princeton University Press.

Said, S. (1993) 'Tragic Argos', in A. H. Sommerstein, S. Halliwell, J. Henderson and B. Zimmermann (eds), *Tragedy, Comedy and the Polis*, Bari, 167–89.

Saller, R. P. (1994) *Patriarchy, Property, and Death in the Roman Family*, Cambridge, Cambridge University Press.

Scarborough, J. (1981) 'Roman Medicine and Public Health', in T. Ogawa (ed.), *Public Health, Proceedings of the 5th International Symposium, Comparative History of Medicine – East and West, 1980*, Tokyo: Saikon.

Scheid, J. (1984) '*Contraria facere*: Renversements et déplacements dans les rites funéraires', *AION Arch. Stor. Ant.* 6, 117–39.

Scheid, J. (1987) 'Les sanctuaires de confins dans la Rome antique. Réalité et permanence d'une representation idéale de l'espace romaine', in *L'Urbs: espace urbain et histoire*, = *Collection de l'École française de Rome* 98, 583–95.

Schilling, R. (1976) 'Le Lares grundules', in *Mélanges. J. Heurgon*, Rome: Ecole française, II 947–60.

Scobie, A. (1986) 'Slums, Sanitation, and Mortality in the Roman world', *Klio* 68, 399–433.

Seaford, R. (1994) *Reciprocity and Ritual*, Oxford.

Sebesta, J. (1997) 'Women's Costume and Feminine Civic Morality in Augustan Rome', in M. Wyke (ed.), *Gender and the Body in Mediterranean Antiquity*, *Gender and History* Special Issue 9/3, 529–41.

Shaw, B. D. (1996) 'Seasons of Death: Aspects of Mortality in Imperial Rome', *JRS* 86, 100–38.

Slack, P. A. (1985) *The Impact of Plague in Tudor and Stuart England*, Oxford: Clarendon Press.

Söllner, A. (1913) *Die hygienischen Anschauungen des römischen Architekten Vitruvius. Ein Beitrag zur antiken Hygiene*, = *Jenaer medizin-historische Beiträge* 4.

Solomon, J. (1985) 'Thucydides and the Recognition of Contagion', *Maia* 37.

Sontag, S. (1979) *Illness as Metaphor*, London: Penguin.

Sontag, S. (1989) *AIDS and its Metaphors*, London: Allen Lane.

Sourvinou Inwood, C. (1995) *'Reading' Greek Death to the End of the Classical Period*, Oxford.

Specter, M. (1994) 'In Russia, Corruption Inflates the Cost of Dying', *New York Times*, 15 November, A 3.

Stewart, P. C. N. (1995) 'Inventing Britain: The Roman Creation and Adaptation of an Image', *Britannia* 26, 1–10.

Strazzulla, M. J. (1989) 'In paludibus moenia constituta: problemi urbanistici di Aquileia in età repubblicana alla luce della documentazione archeologica e delle fonti scritte', *Antichità Altoadriatiche* 35, 187–225.

Strocchia, S. T. (1992) *Death and Ritual in Renaissance Florence*, Baltimore: Johns Hopkins University Press.

Strohmaier, G. (1993) 'Hellenistische Wissenschaft im neugefundenen Galenkommentar zur hippokratischen Schrift "Über die Umwelt" ', in J. Kollesch and D. Nickel (eds), *Galen und das hellenistische Erbe*, Stuttgart: Franz Steiner Verlag.

Stucchi, S. (1965) *L'Agora di Cirene, I.I lati Nord ed Est della Platea Inferiore*, Rome.

Stucchi, S. (1967) *Cirene 1957–67. Un decennio di attivita della Missione Archeologica Italiana a Cirene*, Tripoli.

Stucchi, S. (1975) *Architettura Cirenaica*, Rome.

Susini, G. (1969) 'Fundus Fangonianus', *Stud. Romagn.* 20, 333–9.

Sussman, L. A. (1994) *The Declamations of Calpurnius Flaccus*, Leiden: Brill.

Swain, S. (1994) 'Man and Medicine in Thucydides', *Arethusa* 27, 303–27.

Syme, R. (1983) 'The *pomerium* in the Historia Augusta', in *Historia Augusta Papers*, Oxford: Clarendon Press, 131–45.

Synnott, A. (1993) *The Body Social: Symbolism, Self and Society*, London: Routledge.

Terrenato, N. (1996) 'Murus Romuli', in E. M. Steinby (ed.), *Lexicon Topographicum Urbis Romae* 3, 315–17.

Thaniel, G. (1973) 'Libitina', *LEC* 41 (1973), 46–9.

Thompson, D. J. (1988) *Memphis under the Ptolemies*, Princeton: Princeton University Press.

Todd, M. (1978) *The Walls of Rome*, London, Paul Elek.

Torelli, M. (1982) *Typology and Structure of Roman Historical Reliefs*, Ann Arbor: University of Michigan Press.

Torelli, M. (1992) 'Topografia e iconologia: Arco di Portogallo, *Ara Pacis*, *Ara Providentiae*, *Templum Solis*', *Ostraka* 1, 105–31.

Tortorici, E. (1991) *Argiletum: commercio speculazione edilizia e lotta politica dall'antica topografia di un quartiere di Roma di età repubblicana*, Rome: De Luca.

Toynbee, J. M. C. (1971) *Death and Burial in the Roman World*, London: Thames and Hudson.

Toynbee, J. M. C. and Ward-Perkins, J. (1956) *The Shrine of St. Peter and the Vatican Excavations*, London, New York, Toronto: Longmans, Green and Co.

Traina, G. (1986) 'Paesaggio e "decadenza". La palude nella trasformazione del mondo antico', in A. Giardina (ed.), *Società romana e impero tardoantico*, III, Rome and Bari: Laterza, 711–30.

Traina, G. (1988) *Paludi e bonifiche nel mondo antico*, Rome: L'Erma di Bretschneider.

Uggeri, G. (1990) 'La Via Appia nella politica espansionista di Roma', in S. Quilici Gigli (ed.), *La Via Appia = Quaderni del centro di studio per l'archeologia etrusco-italica* 18, 21–8.

Ullmann, M. (1977) 'Galens Kommentar zu der Schrift *De aere aquis locis*', in R. Joly (ed.), *Actes du Colloque Hippocratique de Mons*, Mons: Université de Mons.

Vanggaard, J. H. (1988) *The Flamen: A Study in the History and Sociology of Roman Religion*, Copenhagen: Museum Tusculanum Press.

Van Hooff, A. (1990) *From Autothanasia to Suicide: Self-Killing in Classical Antiquity*, London: Routledge.

Versnel, H. S. (1970) *Triumphus*, Leiden: Brill.

Ville, G. (1981) *La gladiature en occident des origines à la mort de Domitien*, Rome: École française de Rome (Bibliothèque des Écoles françaises d'Athenes et de Rome).
Visscher, F. de (1963) *Le droit des tombeaux romains*, Florence: Giuffre.
Vitali, L. (1932) *Fonti per la storia della religione cirenaica*, Padova.
Voisin, J. (1984) 'Les Romans, chasseurs de têtes', in *Du châtiment dans la cité. Supplices corporels et peine de mort dans le monde antique*. Collection de l'école Française de Rome 79, 241–93.
Vollmer, F. (1891) 'Laudationum funebrium Romanorum historia', *Jahrbuch für klassischen Phil.*, Suppl. 18, 445–528.
Walde, A. and Hoffman, J. B. (1938) *Lateinische etymologische Wörterbuch*, 3rd edn, Heidelberg: C. Winter.
Wallace-Hadrill, A. (1995) 'Public Honour and Private Shame: The Urban Texture of Pompeii', in T. J. Cornell and K. Lomas (eds), *Urban Society in Roman Italy*, London: UCL Press, 39–62.
Wallace-Hadrill, A. (1998) 'Horti and Hellenisation', in M. Cima and E. La Rocca (eds), *Horti Romani: atti del convegno internazionale, Roma, 4–6 maggio 1995*, Rome: L'Erma di Bretschneider, 1–12.
Wasserstein, A. (1982) 'Galen's Commentary on the Hippocratic Treatise *Airs, Waters, Places* in the Hebrew Translation of Solomon ha-Me'ati', *Proceedings of the Israel Academy of Sciences and Humanities* 6.3, 185–303.
Watson, J. L. (1982) 'Of Flesh and Bones: The Management of Death Pollution in Cantonese Society', in M. Bloch and J. Parry (eds), *Death and the Regeneration of Life*, Cambridge: Cambridge University Press, 155–86.
Watson, J. L. (1988) 'Funeral Specialists in Cantonese Society: Pollution, Performance, and Social Hierarchy', in J. L. Watson and E. Rawski (eds), *Death Ritual in Late Imperial and Modern China*, Berkeley: University of California Press, 109–34.
Weaver, P. R. C. (1972) *Familia Caesaris*, Cambridge: Cambridge University Press.
Weidauer, K. (1954) *Thukydides und die hippokratischen Schriften*, Heidelberg.
Welcker, F. G. (1850) 'Schneiden und Brennen', in *Kleine Schriften* III, Bonn: E. Weber, 209–17.
Wells, C. (1960) 'A Study of Cremation', *Antiquity* 34, 29–37.
Whaley, J. (1981) 'Symbolism for the Survivors: The Disposal of the Dead in Hamburg in the late Seventeenth and Eighteenth Centuries', in J. Whaley (ed.), *Mirrors of Mortality*, New York: St. Martin's Press, 80–105.
White, D. (1998) 'Static versus Reactive Defense: An In-Progress Case study of the Apollonia and Cyrene Fortifications', in G. Paci and S. Marengo (eds), *Cirenaica in Eta Antica. Atti del Convegno Macerata Marzo 1995*, Macerata, 579–612.
White, K. D. (1970) *Roman Farming*, London: Thames and Hudson.
Wiedemann, T. (1992) *Emperors and Gladiators*, London: Routledge.
Williams, F. (1978) *Callimachus' Hymn to Apollo: A Commentary*, Oxford.
Wilson, A. and Levy, H. (1938) *Burial Reform and Funeral Costs*, Oxford.
Winslow, C. E. A. (1943) *The Conquest of Epidemic Disease*, Princeton: Princeton University Press.
Wiseman, T. P. (1970) 'Roman Republican Road-building', *Papers of the British School at Rome* 38, 122–52.
Wiseman, T. P. (1985) *Catullus and His World*, Cambridge: Cambridge University Press.
Wiseman, T. P. (1995) *Remus: A Roman Myth*, Cambridge: Cambridge University Press.
Wiseman, T. P. (1998) 'A Stroll on the Rampart', in M. Cima and E. La Rocca (eds), *Horti Romani. Atti del Convegno Internazionale, BCAR Suppl.* 6, Rome: L'Erma di Bretschneider, 13–22.
Wrigley, E. A. (1987) 'No Death without Birth: The Implications of English Mortality in the Early Modern Period', in R. Porter and A. Wear (eds), *Problems and Methods in the History of Medicine*, London: Croom, 133–50.
Yavetz, Z. (1969) *Plebs and Princeps*, Oxford: Oxford University Press.

Youtie, H. C. (1973) 'Notes on O. Mich. I' (*TAPA* 71 [1940] 650–7), reprinted with addenda in H. C. Youtie, *Scriptiunculae* I, Amsterdam, 90–7, 103–4.
Zanker, P. (1988) *The Power of Images in the Age of Augustus*, trans. A. Shapiro, Ann Arbor: University of Michigan Press.
Zeitlin, F. I. (1990) 'Thebes: Theater of Self and Society in Athenian Drama', in J. Winkler and F. I. Zeitlin (eds), *Nothing to do with Dionysos?*, Princeton, 130–67.
Zevi, F. (1999) 'Sepulcrum Scipionum', in E. M. Steinby (ed.), *Lexicon Topographicum Urbis Romae* 4, 281–5.
Ziolkowski, A. (1992) *The Temples of Mid-Republican Rome and their Historical and Topographical Context*, Rome: L'Erma di Bretschneider.

INDEX